THE · BUSINESS · SIDE · OF · GENERAL · PRACTICE

Making Sense of the Red Book, second edition

NORMAN ELLIS
Under Secretary, British Medical Association

JOHN CHISHOLM
Joint Deputy Chairman and Negotiator,
General Medical Services Committee,
British Medical Association

RADCLIFFE MEDICAL PRESS
OXFORD

British Library Cataloguing in Publication Data
ISBN 1-870905-89-X

Typeset by Advance Typesetting Ltd, Oxfordshire
Printed and bound in Great Britain by Biddles Ltd, Guildford and King's Lynn

Contents

Foreword

THIS book is essential reading for every GP. It is vital that GPs should know what is required under the terms of service of their NHS contract and understand how they should be paid for providing these services. It is equally important to ensure that the information provided to GPs for this purpose is kept up to date. This is why a new edition of the book is required. There have been important changes to the GP contract since its imposition in 1990. This fully revised edition incorporates all these changes and replaces the previous edition, *Making Sense of the New Contract*.

During nineteen years as Secretary of the Liverpool Local Medical Committee, I have seen many cases of GPs unnecessarily experiencing difficulties simply because they have not understood what is required under their contract and how they should be paid for fulfilling these obligations.

This book is a vital reference document to be kept close to hand, which will help you and your staff to avoid these difficulties. Indeed, you may have to chain it down to ensure it can always be found when needed!

IAN BOGLE
Chairman
General Medical Services Committee
British Medical Association

⌶ The Business Side of General Practice

Preface

THIS book is the sequel to *Making Sense of the New Contract*, which was itself the sequel to *Making Sense of the Red Book*. Once again, the text has been extensively rewritten and updated. However, because the authors have been able to approach these texts at a more leisurely pace (a very rare privilege in the world of publishing!) they have taken the opportunity to simplify and clarify much of the original text.

The Statement of Fees and Allowances – the 'Red Book' – has continued to set out the basis on which general practitioners (GPs) are paid, and GPs who wish to understand how they are remunerated need to master its complexities. But the Red Book is daunting and densely legalistic; as a result many doctors are unfamiliar with its contents, just as they are unfamiliar with the details of their contracts with the Family Health Services Authority (FHSA) or Health Board.

This book explains the structure and principles of the Red Book, and although it is sometimes quite complicated in its expression, we hope it is much easier to read than the actual text. We have concentrated on its broad principles and provisions and have tried not to replicate its Byzantine detail. In particular, we have excluded all reference to the changing levels of fees and allowances so that the information contained in this book does not become out of date too quickly.

While the ordering of sections of the SFA is curious and to some extent accidental, with new sections being inserted wherever paragraphs have previously been unallotted, this book attempts to use a more logical sequence. However, a comprehensive index to the Red Book is included, and should allow a reader to gain access to relevant paragraphs of the SFA much more quickly than can be achieved using the outline contents at the front of the Red Book itself. In addition, while paragraphs of the SFA are only referred to in the text of *Making Sense of the Red Book*, second edition, when a reader is specifically directed to the Red Book's detailed provisions, the index to this volume uses the same terms as are used in the separate index to the Red Book, so the reader should easily be able to cross-refer from the text of this book to the detail of the SFA.

Readers must of course remember that only the original text carries the force of law and provides the detail needed for authoritative interpretation and resolution of any dispute as to meaning. The purpose of this book is different – it is to inform the reader of the broad structure of the Red Book and to give an overview of the complexity and range of general practitioners' fees and allowances.

One important matter of interpretation should be mentioned. While broadly speaking the contractual arrangements in Scotland are similar to those in England and Wales, the book does not make specific reference to the differences. The most important such difference is that in Scotland, GPs are in contract with Health Boards, not Family Health Services Authorities.

The history of the Red Book

The Charter for the Family Doctor Service was published by the British Medical Association in March 1965. As a result of the successful negotiations which then took place between the Minister of Health and general practitioner representatives, the Regulations, terms of service and remuneration of GPs were all radically restructured. Regulation 22 of the National Health Service (General Medical and Pharmaceutical Services) Regulations 1966 (now Regulation 34 of the National Health Service [General Medical Services] Regulations 1992) placed upon the Minister of Health (now the Secretary of State for Health) an obligation to publish a statement of payments to doctors, and the Statement of Fees and Allowances was first published in October 1966. Although a surprisingly slim volume compared with the 1993 SFA, its structure and contents will seem surprisingly familiar to anyone acquainted with the modern Red Book. However, it was published as a booklet, and for the first few years amendments were issued to GPs via Executive Council Notices (ECNs). As a result, GPs soon found it hard to be certain of their entitlements.

Therefore in 1972 the loose-leaf, ring-bound version of the SFA was introduced, that is now so familiar as the Red Book. Subsequent amendments have been published as replacement or additional pages that allow a GP to maintain an up-to-date version of the Statement. The importance of ensuring that all SFA amendments are received and promptly incorporated into the Red Book cannot be emphasized too strongly. An out-of-date text is misleading and can lead to both false and overlooked claims.

At the end of 1989, a new Red Book was issued to all GPs, for the first time since 1972. This ensured that all GPs had a properly ordered, up-to-date Statement, defining the fees and allowances payable from 1 April 1990 under the 1990 contract.

In the past, amendments to the Red Book have been published at a rate of some nine a year, but often these have been confined to changes in one paragraph of the SFA, and have been quite brief. Since the introduction of the 1990 contract there have been 14 sets of amendments, many of them significant and extensive; these are listed in Appendix 4 for ease of reference.

Particularly significant amendments have been made to protect confidential personal information when claims are made for minor surgery session fees and cervical cytology target payments; to alter the arrangements for the direct reimbursement of trainee practitioners' medical defence organization subscriptions; to reimburse directly a wider range of computing costs; to amend the procedures for representations to the Secretary of State; to change target payment calculations from an individual to a partnership list basis; to improve the rural practice payments scheme; to introduce new health promotion arrangements; to amend the arrangements for payment of higher rate night visit fees; and to pay GPs for *Haemophilus influenzae b* immunization.

As a result of these and other changes, the text of this book has been substantially revised.

The Business Side of General Practice

The original idea for a simple guide to the Statement of Fees and Allowances came from Stuart Carne. He discussed his proposal with Andrew Bax, the Managing Director of Radcliffe Medical Press, and from that initial suggestion has grown the idea for a series of books entitled The Business Side of General Practice. *Making Sense of the Red Book* was published in 1989, *Making Sense of the New Contract* in 1990, and this present volume is essentially a radically revised and rewritten version of the 1990 book.

The readers of these books are not only general practitioners, but also trainee practitioners, doctors' professional advisers and their practice staff – particularly practice managers, and also receptionists and all those who help to run the doctor's office.

With such a readership in mind, an Editorial Board for The Business Side of General Practice was formed. It deliberately includes representatives of both the elected members and the secretariat of the General Medical Services Committee of the British Medical Association; a representative of the Royal College of General Practitioners; a Local Medical Committee secretary; a Family Health Services Authority general manager; and representatives of the Association of Health Centre and Practice Administrators and the Association of Medical Secretaries, Practice Administrators and Receptionists. As a result, experts on terms and conditions of service, on training and education, and on the needs of readers, have been brought together to share their experience.

Acknowledgements

The first two versions of this book were edited by one of us, John Chisholm, and written by the other, Norman Ellis, together with three authors with experience of administering FPCs and managing FHSAs: Paul Bates, Tim Brown and Bill Robinson. We are very grateful to them for the great contribution they made to those earlier books, which has formed much of the foundation to this volume.

We also wish to thank the Editorial Board for their helpful comments on the text, and particularly Stuart Carne for inspiring The Business Side of General Practice series of books. We are indebted to Ian Bogle for writing the foreword; Andrew Lockhart-Mirans of Hempsons Solicitors and Chris Hughes, solicitor and Head of Legal Services at the BMA, for their help with the list of Regulations; Liz Housden, Assistant Secretary at the BMA, for her guidance about GPs' remuneration; and Bill Roberts, former Assistant Secretary at the Department of Health and Social Security, who devised the loose-leaf format of the Red Book and has informed us about the history of the SFA.

Above all, we are grateful to Andrew Bax. His enthusiasm and energy, and the high production standards of Radcliffe Medical Press, have been crucial in producing what we hope will be a valuable and practical guide to all who wish to understand the content of the Red Book.

NORMAN ELLIS
JOHN CHISHOLM
June 1993

1 Independent contractor status

AN independent contractor is a self-employed person who has entered into a contract for services with another party. This contract for services is fundamentally different from the contract of service which governs an employee–employer relationship. A key test, often used to distinguish between these two types of contract, relates to the question of 'control'. Generally, the more control A exercises over B's work, the more likely A is to be the employer and B the employee. Thus, if A can tell B not only what job to do but how it is to be done, A has sufficient control to make him B's employer.

However, if the exercise of control is much more diffuse, such that the person doing the work is not told how to do it, the contract is for services and the relationship is between what is confusingly known in legal terminology as 'the principal party' and 'an independent contractor'. Obviously, this test is crude and there are borderline cases, but the status of the National Health Service (NHS) general practitioner (GP) as an independent contractor has not been seriously questioned in the past. As an independent contractor a GP should not be told by the Family Health Services Authority (FHSA) or Health Board how to practise. FHSAs and Health Boards should seek to persuade and advise, not direct or control.

The character of British general practice has been strongly influenced by the independent contractor status of its practitioners. The remuneration system, the organization of practices into partnerships, together with the medico-political institutions that enable GPs to exercise professional self-government, demonstrate this influence.

As independent contractors, GPs exercise discretion and freedom in how they run their practices. This autonomy carries with it the administrative and financial responsibility for running the business itself and also responsibility for the clinical services provided. These responsibilities include providing premises, staff and equipment. If GPs were health authority employees (like hospital consultants), the authority would be responsible for providing these resources.

The main advantages of an independent contractor service are its flexibility and adaptability, and the fact that it can offer a more personalized model of care. It also provides opportunities for innovation and diversity without interference, and gives patients scope for choice. Disadvantages may be apparent if the standards of service are allowed to vary widely. Those who are responsible for administering GPs' contracts sometimes see this arrangement as untidy and unsatisfactory, because the means of control available to an employer are lacking.

No other occupation (apart from the other Family Health Services contractor professions – dentists, chemists and opticians) has this unique partnership with the State, or with the public. In current parlance, general practice is the original 'privatized' sector of the NHS. GPs in other Western developed economies, together with most other professionals, such as dentists, lawyers, architects, surveyors and accountants, are also independent contractors. In the United Kingdom, GPs have jealously guarded their independent contractor status ever since Lloyd George's national insurance scheme was introduced in 1911. The profession supported the idea of a State-funded medical scheme, but it was adamantly opposed to a salaried service; it recognized that the loss of independent contractor status would undermine the freedom of doctors to practise without State interference and ultimately put patient care at risk. GPs feared that government would seek to direct them in their day-to-day treatment of patients. This commitment to the independent contractor status underlies the policy of the Conference of Representatives of Local Medical Committees (LMCs).

The implementation of the new contractual arrangements is changing the relationship between individual GPs and the FHSA. New controls are being exercised by FHSAs over the work of GPs. GPs are now required to report annually to the FHSA giving information on their practice population and on prescribing arrangements, and also have to provide a more detailed statement of the hours they are available to patients for surgery consultations, clinics and home visits.

Additionally, the new arrangements specify more precisely the services GPs are required to provide for patients. The terms of service have been amended to make clear that health promotion and illness prevention fall within the remit of general medical services. The services that are required of the GP are spelt out in some detail, specifying which procedures should be undertaken and which patients should be offered which services.

During the debate on the imposition of the new arrangements, the question was raised as to whether the new Regulations and terms of service were incompatible with the GP's status as an independent contractor. Whilst there can be no doubt that greater control is now exercised over the work of the GP, both the Government and the General Medical Services Committee (GMSC) of the British Medical Association (BMA) are agreed that the GP should continue to work as an independent contractor: indeed, in a joint statement from the Department of Health and the GMSC the Secretary of State for Health 'confirmed that the independent contractor status of GPs would not be affected'.

However, the question of whether GPs are independent contractors is not something which can be resolved by the declared wishes of the two parties directly concerned. It depends ultimately upon whether the control exercised by FHSAs is sufficiently diffuse to justify retention of the independent contractor status.

In spite of the increased accountability required under the new contract – and the increased powers of FHSAs – there should be no doubt that GPs continue to work as independent contractors. The old contract also contained detailed specification of certain clinical tasks (such as those relating to the provision of maternity care) and these have never been regarded as being incompatible with the independent contractor status.

2 How GPs' pay is determined

THE Doctors' and Dentists' Review Body was set up in 1960, as a consequence of the recommendations of a Royal Commission known as the Pilkington Commission. Its remit is to recommend to the Prime Minister the levels of remuneration of doctors (and dentists) working in the NHS.

The Pilkington Commission was concerned to ensure that doctors' pay should not be used as a means of regulating pay movements in the economy; it wanted to see their pay removed from the political arena. The Commission considered various options, including direct negotiations, collective bargaining through Whitley machinery (used by most health service employees), and arbitration. It recommended an independent review body and laid down its ground rules (*see* Box 2.1).

Box 2.1: The Review Body's ground rules

- the Review Body's main task was to exercise 'good judgement'
- although the government had the ultimate power to decide, Review Body recommendations must only be rejected by government very rarely, and for most obviously compelling reasons
- government should deal with Review Body recommendations promptly
- the remuneration of doctors should be determined primarily, though not exclusively, by external comparison with other professions and similarly qualified employees
- doctors should not be used by governments as part of their machinery for regulating the economy; they have a right to be treated fairly and the profession should assist the Review Body by willingly providing information about earnings
- doctors' earnings should not be determined according to short-term supply and demand considerations

---

How the Review Body system works

Although the Review Body is willing to receive evidence from any interested party, it concentrates on evidence from a few key sources (*see* Box 2.2).

Both sides, the professions and the Health Departments, normally submit written evidence to the Review Body on the same day, and also exchange evidence. This means that each side prepares its evidence 'in the dark', without sight of the other evidence.

> **Box 2.2: Main sources of evidence to the Review Body**
>
> - written evidence from the medical profession, prepared by the BMA
> - written evidence from the dental profession
> - written evidence from the Health Departments
> - joint written evidence agreed between the profession and the Health Departments, usually dealing with matters already agreed in negotiation
> - jointly agreed statistical information, e.g. evidence on GPs' earnings and expenses
> - independent evidence prepared by the Review Body's secretariat, (Office of Manpower Economics) e.g. various surveys conducted at the request of the Review Body

The next stage involves oral hearings. The Review Body meets each side, using the occasion to clarify any subject raised in the written evidence or to discuss other points of concern. The parties will also use the oral sessions to emphasize or update any matter in their written evidence.

Having considered all the evidence, the Review Body reports in confidence to the Prime Minister. Further time usually elapses before the report is published and the government announces its decision on whether to implement the recommendations.

General practitioners' remuneration

As independent contractors, GPs are paid a gross income by the NHS, out of which they meet practice expenses, including items such as staff salaries, the cost of surgery premises, and motoring expenses. The GPs' payment system is based on a principle known as 'cost plus'; the payments received are intended both to cover their expenses and to provide a net income.

The Review Body recommends what it considers to be an appropriate level of net income for GPs, and taking account of this recommendation the government decides upon the average level of income of all GPs. In fact, individual GPs receive greatly varying amounts depending upon the particular circumstances of their practices; expenses and list sizes differ and GPs provide a varying range of services. Virtually all GPs earn either more or less than the average; it is exceptionally rare to discover a GP whose earnings coincide exactly with the average figure.

The component for expenses should be added to net income. All expenses incurred by GPs in providing general medical services are paid back to the profession in full: some are paid directly to the individual GP actually incurring them (these are known as directly reimbursed expenses); the remainder of GPs' expenses are reimbursed indirectly on an averaging basis through fees and allowances. Thus, the exact amount an individual GP receives in indirectly reimbursed expenses will not, except by pure chance, equal expenditure, and in practice, there will be a strong incentive for a GP to economize on his or her own practice expenses.

Although this way of dealing with GPs' expenses is complex and can lead to anomalies and inequalities, it does recognize the independent contractor status of the family doctor, which is fundamentally different from that of salaried colleagues employed elsewhere in the NHS. A possible alternative approach could have been to require each GP to submit to the FHSA a monthly or quarterly claim for expenses, which it would check (and no doubt question on occasion). If this arrangement had been adopted, the profession would have given up its independence to choose how to run its practices. The significance of this is not always recognized by those who call for increased direct reimbursement.

It has been argued that because around half of practice expenses are repaid indirectly through fees and allowances, irrespective of what is spent, the less an individual GP spends on the practice the greater will be his or her profits. Although there is some truth in this view, it does not represent the whole picture. GPs are directly reimbursed for part of the cost of providing many of the most costly items (for example, surgery premises and practice staff). A GP who chooses to underfund his or her practice will find it lagging behind other practices in the services it can offer; it will not be as attractive to new patients and patients currently on the list may opt to change to other practices in the neighbourhood. A contrary and more positive view needs to be stated. If those GPs who are unwilling to invest in their own practices would overcome their reticence, the profession as a whole would benefit through the indirect reimbursement system and general practice would become more capital intensive. For example, if every GP decided to invest in an ECG machine, under the present system the NHS would have no option but to fund this investment through the indirect reimbursement scheme.

An explanation of how GPs' expenditure on defence body subscriptions is indirectly reimbursed illustrates this point. Almost every GP subscribes to a medical defence body, and traditionally the amount each GP pays has been broadly similar. Thus, every GP is faced with an equivalent level of expenditure. These subscriptions have been paid ever since the present GPs' remuneration structure was established in the 1960s and therefore this expenditure is built into the system. The Review Body is aware that defence body subscriptions must be paid and that these have increased rapidly. It is therefore able to make provision for this expenditure in its estimates of GPs' expenses, including an element to take account of anticipated increases in the subscription rate. As almost all GPs pay this subscription, it is reimbursed through fees and allowances (and because future increases have been taken into account) at close to the prevailing rate.

Expenditure that is fully and directly reimbursed

Certain practice expenses are reimbursed directly to each GP. However, while the direct reimbursement is treated as practice income, the expenditure is claimed against income tax. The GP's tax return may be used to calculate those expenses to be reimbursed indirectly through the fees and allowances. Direct reimbursements may be full or partial. Those items reimbursed directly and fully are listed in Box 2.3.

Box 2.3: Items of GP expenditure that are reimbursed directly and fully

- surgery rent and rates, water rates, water meter installation and charges, and refuse collection charges
- employer's national insurance contributions in respect of GP trainees and some practice staff
- employer's pension contributions in respect of GP trainees and certain approved schemes for practice staff
- net ingredient cost plus VAT of drugs dispensed under the drug tariff

---

Full direct reimbursement of all of a GP's spending under any heading occurs only when the government or some public agency has direct control over its costs, as is the case with national insurance contributions. Likewise, the GP receives full direct reimbursement of surgery rent if the rent is approved by a district valuer. Dispensing doctors are repaid 100% of the cost of drugs they prescribe and dispense, because drug prices are effectively controlled by government. A GP trainer receives full reimbursement for the trainee's salary and car allowance and employer's national insurance and superannuation contributions, because again all these costs are within the control of government.

Expenditure that is partially directly reimbursed

The most common partial direct reimbursement is the refund of practice staff salaries. Examples of allowances with maximum or fixed ceilings include those relating to the employment of an assistant, employment of a locum to cover a GP's absence because of sickness, maternity or study leave, and payments made under the doctors' retainer scheme.

The imposition of cash limits on the funds available to FHSAs for direct reimbursements means that the percentage of the salary refunded in respect of future staff appointments may differ from the fixed rate of 70% reimbursement paid under the former ancillary staff scheme. FHSAs can now exercise discretion in determining the level of direct reimbursement, and thus it may vary from zero to 100%.

A scheme for the partial direct reimbursement of computing costs was introduced in 1990, and provides for the direct payment of a proportion of the costs of purchase, leasing, upgrading and maintenance of a computer system.

Indirectly reimbursed expenditure

As described above, each year the Review Body estimates on the basis of a survey of tax returns how much GPs as a whole will spend on providing general medical services, and calculates an average figure for each GP's indirect expenses after taking into account the total expenditure on direct reimbursements. This figure for average indirect expenses is added to the level of pre-tax pay which the Review Body considers appropriate for GPs to earn, known as net remuneration, and the resulting figure becomes the gross remuneration. The various fees and allowances that comprise a GP's pay are then adjusted so that during the year they yield for the average GP the total gross and net remuneration which the Review Body has deemed appropriate.

This exercise is complex, and because the 'targets' set by the Review Body are not always met, any under- or over-payment is allowed for in subsequent years. As the Department of Health is apprised of how much has been paid to GPs after the end of a financial year, it is not difficult to compare the level of average gross pay received with the original target. Average net pay is more difficult to calculate because this depends upon an analysis of income tax returns.

Because GPs wish to obtain tax relief, they inform the Inland Revenue of the expenditure they have incurred in providing general medical services. This is the key source of information for estimating GP expenses. Once a year, the Inland Revenue provides anonymized information relating to a sample of GPs' accounts. It includes all personal, professional and partnership expenses.

General practitioner accounts

As the level of expenses to be reimbursed is always based upon samples of income tax returns, it is vital that all GPs record their expenses correctly.

For revenue items, GPs should enter the full amounts of both directly and indirectly reimbursed expenses, including those items that may not appear in cash books, bank statements or cheque books. Examples include those payments made by FHSAs directly to health authorities or other bodies on behalf of the practice, such as health centre rents, waste disposal charges and levies. The practice of 'netting off' expenses against matching income must be avoided; failure to include expenses, however small, reduces the funding available to the profession as a whole.

Where capital items are concerned – for example, computers and equipment purchased from the practice fund management allowance – standard accounting practice should be followed. Usually this will involve depreciating assets net of any Government grant received.

3 GPs' terms of service

GPs working in the NHS have a contract with the FHSA to provide general medical services to their NHS patients. It is important to note that this contract is with the FHSA not the patient, in contrast to most other countries where doctors have a direct contractual commitment to patients. Given this independent contractor status with a statutory authority within a publicly funded health service, it is not surprising to find that the NHS GP's contract has been enshrined in legislation, the NHS (General Medical Services) Regulations (*see* Table 3.1).

The regulations, which include the GP's terms of service, provide the legal framework within which the business of NHS general practice is conducted. Because these regulations are laid down by Parliament their style and format inevitably reflect their parliamentary origin; this makes them difficult for a layman to comprehend, and the difficulty is compounded by the publication of amendments. The Regulations have been amended on several occasions; as many as a dozen amendments have been issued since 1 April 1985 following the introduction of the limited list of NHS drugs. However, in November 1989 major amendments were introduced to implement new contractual arrangements with effect from 1 April 1990, and each GP was sent a copy of the amended terms of service. In April 1992 a completely revised and consolidated version of the Regulations was made, and a copy of this was also sent to each GP. This new version rationalized the arrangement of the Regulations and no longer includes the Pharmaceutical Services Regulations.

Therefore, at the same time as the consolidated GMS Regulations were published, consolidated Pharmaceutical Services Regulations were also distributed. They included regulations governing the provision of pharmaceutical services by doctors, and how rurality is determined in relation to doctor and chemist dispensing.

There is an understandable reluctance to provide a definitive explanatory guide to the Regulations. Since they carry the force of law, any dispute about their application or meaning can be resolved only by reference to the original text. Each copy of the Regulations, and subsequent amending Regulations, is accompanied by an official explanatory note, but it is always stated that this note does not form part of the Regulations as such. Nevertheless, a doctor needs to know what is required to fulfil the contract with the FHSA. In part, this knowledge is acquired from colleagues and partners, and the FHSA. Advice from the General Medical Services Committee (GMSC) and from the Local Medical Committee (LMC), together with information in the

Table 3.1. National Health Service (General Medical Services) Regulations 1992

The Regulations are in seven parts:

I   General: citation and commencement; interpretation; scope and terms of service

II   The Medical List: medical list; applying for inclusion or succession to a vacancy; amending of or withdrawing from it; removal from it; local directory of family doctors

III   Medical Practices Committee: membership; reports; procedure for filling vacancies; certifying sale of goodwill not involved

IV   General Medical Services other than Child Health Surveillance Services, Contraceptive Services, Maternity Medical Services and Minor Surgery Services: describes how patients apply to be on a doctor's list; how patients are assigned to doctors; the limits on list size; how patients transfer to another doctor; how patients are removed from a doctor's list; arrangements for temporary residents; temporary arrangements for running a practice

V   Child Health Surveillance Services, Contraceptive Services, Maternity Medical Services and Minor Surgery Services: explains the separate lists for each of these services and how these services are obtained

VI   Payments to doctors: requires the Secretary of State to publish the Statement of Fees and Allowances (the Red Book) and to pay doctors accordingly

VII   Miscellaneous: whether a substance is a drug; appointment of medical advisers; guidance to doctors.

medical journals, all help to familiarize the doctor with the Regulations and terms of service. Such advice should help a GP to be aware of current issues concerning their interpretation and application.

Every GP should have access to a copy of the principal Regulations and any amending Regulations. Copies are distributed by FHSAs and additional copies may be obtained from them. Nevertheless, many practices rarely refer to the Regulations and, if a difficulty ever arises, a GP usually seeks advice from his or her LMC secretary or FHSA general manager.

Alleged breaches of the terms of service by a GP are normally dealt with by the Medical Service Committee (MSC) of the FHSA with which the GP is in contract. A separate set of Regulations deals with the MSC procedure (Statutory Instrument No 455 [1974], the National Health Service [Service Committees and Tribunal] Regulations 1974, and subsequent amendments).

It is essential that all GPs are aware of the Regulations because they contain the terms of service which form the basis of their NHS contracts. They should be referred to if any problems arise, and if there is any doubt about their meaning GPs should seek advice from their LMC.

The commentary below focuses on the main aspects of a GP's terms of service; it should help GPs to understand schedule 2 of the Regulations which contains those terms of service. This selective commentary is not a substitute for the original text and should not be quoted if any problem arises.

The 1990 contract

Amendments to the Regulations arising from the 1990 contract introduced into GPs' terms of service important new elements of the contract which would previously have been included in the Statement of Fees and Allowances (SFA or Red Book); these include those relating to the arrangements for providing child health surveillance and minor surgery services, and screening elderly and newly registered patients. By including these parts of the contract in the Regulations rather than in the SFA, the government has ensured they are subject to Parliamentary rather than administrative control, thus keeping them firmly in the public arena and preventing them from being modified without the explicit consent of Parliament.

The GPs' terms of service

Professional judgement

When a GP has to decide what, if any, professional action needs to be taken under the terms of service, in reaching such a decision, he or she is not expected to exercise a higher degree of skill, knowledge and care than may reasonably be expected of GPs generally. Any GP who wants clarification on a matter involving professional judgement should consult his or her LMC secretary or defence body. The same general principle also applies to GPs providing child health surveillance or maternity medical or minor surgery services; in each area the level of skill, knowledge and care expected is that which may reasonably be expected of any doctor included in the appropriate list.

Patients

The terms of service specify those categories of persons who are a GP's patients (*see* Table 3.2). Most are self-evident. However, it is important to note that if a patient seeking treatment claims to be on a GP's list but fails to produce a medical card, and the GP has reasonable doubts about the claim, the GP should nevertheless provide treatment but is entitled to ask for a fee. If the patient is subsequently able to prove to the FHSA that he or she is on the GP's list, the fee has to be refunded.

Table 3.2. Who are a GP's patients?

The main categories are:

- persons on the GP's list

- persons whom the GP has accepted or agreed to accept on the list and who have not been notified to him or her by the FHSA as having ceased to be on it

- for a limited period of up to 14 days, persons the GP has refused to accept on to the list, if they live in the practice area and are not on the list of another doctor in the same area, or persons the GP has refused to accept as temporary residents

- persons who have been assigned to the GP under Regulation 21

- for a limited period, persons about whom the GP has been notified that an application has been made for assignment to him or her

- persons accepted as temporary residents

- persons eligible for acceptance as temporary residents whom the GP agrees to take a smear from, vaccinate or immunize

- persons to whom the GP is requested to give treatment which is immediately required owing to an accident or other emergency at any place in the practice area, or any persons to whom the GP agrees on request to give treatment which is immediately required owing to an accident or other emergency at any place in the FHSA locality, provided that there is no other doctor at the time otherwise obliged and available to give treatment

- persons for whom the GP is acting as a deputy to another doctor under the terms of service

- persons whom the GP has been appointed to treat temporarily

- persons for whom the GP has undertaken to provide child health surveillance or minor surgery services

- women for whom the GP has undertaken to provide contraceptive or maternity medical services

- persons whose own doctor has been relieved of responsibility for them during hours arranged with the FHSA, for whom the GP has accepted responsibility during those hours.

Providing child health surveillance and minor surgery

GPs on the FHSA list may provide to a patient on their list (or on a partner's list or the list of a GP with whom they are in group practice) child health surveillance and/or minor surgery services, and may be paid for these services if included on the relevant list of the FHSA.

A GP who has agreed to provide child health surveillance services should:

- provide those services listed in Table 3.3 below (except for any examination the parent refuses to allow) until the child attains the age five
- maintain the records specified in Table 3.4
- provide the health authority with the information specified in Table 3.5.

Table 3.3.   Child health surveillance services

These services comprise:

(a)   the monitoring:
(i)   by the consideration of information concerning the child received by or on behalf of the doctor, and
(ii)   on any occasion when the child is examined or observed by or on behalf of the doctor (whether pursuant to sub-paragraph (b) or otherwise) of the health, well-being and physical, mental and social development (all of which characteristics are referred to as 'development') of the child while under the age of five years with a view to detecting any deviations from normal development
(b)   the examination of the child by or on behalf of the doctor on so many occasions and at such intervals as shall have been agreed between the FHSA and the health authority in whose district the child resides ('the relevant health authority') for the purpose of the provision of child health surveillance services generally in that district.

Table 3.4.   Child health surveillance services: records

The GP should keep an accurate record of:

(a)   the development of the child under the age of five years, compiled as soon as is reasonably practicable following the first examination and, where appropriate, amended following each subsequent examination, and
(b)   the responses (if any) to offers made to the child's parent for the child to undergo any examination.

Table 3.5.   Child health surveillance services

The GP should provide the health authority with the following information:

(a)   a statement, to be prepared and dispatched to the relevant health authority as soon as is reasonably practicable following any examination, of the procedures undertaken in the course of that examination and of the doctor's findings in relation to each such procedure
(b)   such further information regarding the development of the child while under the age of five years as the relevant health authority may request.

GPs who have agreed to provide minor surgery services should:

- offer to provide any of the procedures listed in Table 3.6 as appropriate
- if providing minor surgery services to a patient not on their list, inform the patient's GP in writing of the outcome of the procedure.

Table 3.6. Minor surgery procedures

Injections	intra-articular
	peri-articular
	varicose veins
	haemorrhoids
Aspirations	joints
	cysts
	bursae
	hydrocele
Incisions	abscesses
	cysts
	thrombosed piles
Excisions	sebaceous cysts
	lipoma
	skin lesions for histology
	intradermal naevi, papillomata, dermatofibromata and similar conditions
	warts
	removal of toe nails (partial or complete)
Curette cautery and cryocautery	warts and verrucae
	other skin lesions (e.g. molluscum contagiosum)
Other	removal of foreign bodies
	nasal cautery

Terminating responsibility for patients

GPs may apply to the FHSA to have any person removed from their list. This takes effect on the date of acceptance by, or assignment to, another doctor, or on the eighth day after applying to the FHSA, whichever is sooner. However, if a GP is treating the person when removal would normally take effect, the FHSA should be informed and removal will take effect only on the eighth day after the FHSA receives notification that the patient no longer requires treatment, or upon acceptance by another doctor, whichever occurs first.

This right to remove a patient has to be set against the duty of an FHSA to assign a patient to a GP when the patient is unable to obtain acceptance voluntarily. In an area served by only one GP, this severely restricts a doctor's right to remove.

A GP may agree with a patient to stop providing her with maternity medical services (MMS) and, failing agreement, may apply for permission to terminate the arrangement. The FHSA may agree to this after considering the views of either party and consulting the LMC. If the GP stops providing MMS the patient must be told so that she can make alternative arrangements with another doctor.

A GP's agreement to provide child health surveillance services may be terminated:

- by either the parent or the doctor
- if the child has been removed from the doctor's list (or his or her partner's list or that of a doctor with whom he or she is associated in a group practice)
- if the parent fails to respond to an invitation to arrange for the child to attend for examination within 42 days.

If the GP's undertaking to provide these services has ceased to be effective he or she should inform the FHSA and, where appropriate, also inform the patient.

Services to patients

GPs are required to provide for their patients all necessary and appropriate personal medical services of the type usually provided by GPs. These should be provided at the practice premises or, if the condition of the patient requires, where the patient was living when accepted as a patient, or elsewhere in the practice area. The GP is not required to visit or treat the patient at any other place, but care has to be taken to ensure that neither the GP nor a member of his or her staff implies there is a willingness to visit at an address outside the practice area. If this should happen, the GP may be bound by a duty to visit.

There is no obligation to provide contraceptive services, child health surveillance services, minor surgery services, or, except in an emergency, maternity services, unless the GP has previously agreed to do so.

The doctor should, unless prevented by an emergency, attend and treat any patient who comes for treatment at the places and during the hours approved by the FHSA, other than a patient who attends when an appointment system is in operation and has not made an appointment. In these circumstances the doctor may decline to see the patient during that surgery period, providing the patient's health would not be put at risk and the patient is offered an appointment to attend within a reasonable time. GPs should take all reasonable steps to ensure that a consultation is not so deferred without their knowledge.

The Regulations specify in detail certain services a GP is required to provide; these include:

- giving advice, as appropriate, to a patient about the patient's general health, and in particular about diet, exercise, the use of tobacco, the consumption of alcohol and the misuse of drugs and solvents
- offering patients consultations and, where appropriate, physical examinations to identify or reduce the risk of disease or injury
- offering patients, as appropriate, vaccination or immunization against measles, mumps, rubella, pertussis, poliomyelitis, diphtheria and tetanus
- arranging for patients to be referred to other NHS services
- giving advice to enable patients to obtain help from a local authority social services department.

Newly registered patients

If a patient has been accepted on to a GP's list (or assigned to it) the patient should be offered a consultation within 28 days to:

- obtain details of the patient's medical history, and when relevant that of his or her family, relating to:
  - (i) illnesses, immunizations, allergies, hereditary conditions, medication and tests carried out for breast or cervical cancer
  - (ii) social factors (including employment, housing and family circumstances) which may affect health
  - (iii) lifestyle factors (including diet, exercise, use of tobacco, consumption of alcohol, and misuse of drugs and solvents) which may affect health
  - (iv) the current state of the patient's health
- physically examine the patient:
  - (i) measuring height, weight and blood pressure
  - (ii) taking and analysing a urine sample to identify the presence of albumin and glucose
- record in the patient's notes the results of this examination
- assess whether and to what extent personal medical services should be provided to the patient
- offer to discuss with the patient (or the parent of a child patient) the conclusions of the consultation as to the state of the patient's health.

When offering a consultation for this purpose, the GP should:

- provide a written invitation − or if the initial invitation is made orally, provide written confirmation

- record in the patient's medical records the date of each invitation and whether it was accepted
- where, as a result of making the invitation, the doctor becomes aware that a patient is no longer residing at the address given in the records, inform the FHSA.

A GP is not required to offer a consultation to a newly registered patient if:

- he or she is a restricted services principal (i.e. a principal who has only undertaken to provide child health services, contraceptive services, maternity medical services, or minor surgery services, or some combination of these)
- the patient is a child under the age of five
- the patient was, immediately before joining the list, on that of a partner and had already had a consultation of this kind during the previous 12 months.

If a GP assumes responsibility for a list of patients on succession to a vacant practice, or becomes responsible for a sizeable number of new patients over a short period, the GP can ask the FHSA to defer the obligation to offer these consultations.

Patients aged 75 years and over

The GP should offer each patient a consultation and a domiciliary visit (which may be combined) to assess whether the patient requires treatment. This offer should be made no later than 1 April 1994 to any patient over the age of 75 years on the GP's list on 31 March 1993. For a patient who attains the age of 75 on or after 1 April 1993, the domiciliary visit and consultation should be offered within 12 months of the patient's 75th birthday. If a patient joins a GP's list and is already aged 75, the offer should be made within 12 months. The GP should make the offer in writing (or confirm it in writing if made orally) and keep a record of the date of the invitation and whether it was accepted.

The doctor should record anything which appears to be affecting the patient's general health, including:

- sensory functions
- mobility
- mental condition
- physical condition including continence
- social environment
- use of medicines.

The GP should also record the findings of the domiciliary visit. After the domiciliary consultation, the GP should offer to discuss with the patient any conclusions that have been drawn.

Absences, deputies, assistants and partners

Normally, a GP should give treatment personally. However, in the case of general medical services other than maternity medical services, child health surveillance and minor surgery services, the GP is under no obligation to do so if reasonable steps are taken to ensure continuity of treatment by another doctor acting as a deputy, irrespective of whether the other doctor is a partner or an assistant. In addition, if it is reasonable to delegate the clinical treatment to a person whom the GP has authorized and who is competent to carry it out (e.g. a qualified nurse), the GP may do so.

A doctor on the obstetric list should not, without the FHSA's consent, employ a deputy or assistant to provide maternity services who is not (or is not qualified by experience to be) included on the obstetric list. However, this does not apply in an obstetric emergency.

As for child health surveillance services, a GP who has agreed to provide these may employ a deputy or an assistant on a child health surveillance list, or with the FHSA's agreement another deputy or assistant. A GP who has agreed to provide minor surgery services may employ a deputy or assistant who is on a minor surgery list.

In general, GPs are responsible for the acts and omissions of any doctors acting as their deputies, whether the deputy is a partner or an assistant. GPs are similarly responsible for any person they employ or who acts on their behalf. **However, a GP is not responsible under the terms of service for the acts and omissions of a deputy who is on the list of same FHSA.**

The FHSA should be informed of any standing deputizing arrangements unless the deputy is the GP's assistant or is already on the FHSA's list, and carries out these arrangements at the premises where the doctor normally practises. If GPs are absent for more than a week, the FHSA should be told who is responsible for the practice during their absence.

Before entering into any arrangement with a deputizing service, GPs should obtain the FHSA's consent. When giving consent, the FHSA may impose conditions to ensure that the arrangements are adequate, but must consult the LMC before refusing consent or imposing conditions. The FHSA is required to review any consent given or conditions imposed in consultation with the LMC, and may withdraw consent or alter the conditions. A GP may appeal to the Secretary of State against a refusal or withdrawal of consent, or the imposition or variation of conditions.

GPs should take reasonable steps to satisfy themselves that any doctor employed as a deputy or assistant is not disqualified from inclusion on the FHSA's list. The GP should tell the FHSA the name of any assistant employed and when this employment ends. A doctor should not employ one or more assistants for more than three months in a period of 12 months without FHSA consent. The FHSA may review and withdraw its consent, but before refusing or withdrawing consent, the FHSA must consult the LMC. (A GP may appeal to the Medical Practices Committee (MPC) against refusal or withdrawal of consent.) If consent is withdrawn, the decision will not take effect for a month; but if an appeal is made to the MPC against withdrawal and it dismisses the appeal, the withdrawal takes effect from a date determined by the MPC, not less than one month after the date of dismissal. (A doctor acting as a deputy can treat patients at places and times other than those arranged by the GP for whom he or she is deputizing although regard must be given to the convenience of the patients.)

Arrangements at practice premises

The GP should provide adequate accommodation at the practice premises 'having regard to the circumstances of his practice' and is required, on receiving a written request from the FHSA, to allow the premises to be visited at any reasonable time by a representative of either the FHSA or LMC, or both.

If a GP intends to run an appointment system (or succeeds to or joins a practice where one is already running) the FHSA should be told about the system he or she proposes to operate or any proposal to discontinue it.

With certain important exceptions, a GP should not, without the consent of the FHSA (or, on appeal, the MPC), practise at premises previously used by another doctor whose practice has been declared vacant and to whose practice a successor has been or is to be appointed.

The GP should not without the consent of the FHSA (or, on appeal, the MPC) start to practise in any premises within one year of their having ceased to be occupied or used for the purpose of practice by another doctor who within one month of such cessation begins practising at a group practice premises, as a member of a group, or at a health centre less than three miles away from the original premises. (This does not apply if the former occupant gives written consent for another doctor to use the premises.)

Employees

Before employing any member of staff, the GP should ensure that the person is suitably qualified and competent to carry out the required duties. In particular, the doctor should take account of the employee's academic and vocational qualifications, training and previous experience. The GP should also offer the employee reasonable training opportunities.

Availability to patients

Any GP should normally be available at times and places approved by the FHSA and inform patients of his or her availability. In general, the FHSA will not approve any application unless satisfied that the times proposed are such that the GP is normally available:

- 42 weeks in any period of 12 months
- during not less than 26 hours in any such week
- on five days in any such week
- with hours of availability which are likely to be convenient to patients.

There are important exceptions to this basic requirement:

- a GP may seek to be normally available for 26 hours over a four day week, if he or she is involved in health-related activities other than providing general medical services to his or her patients (*see* Table 3.7 overleaf, for a broad definition of health related activities). But the four day availability will not be approved by the FHSA if it considers that the effectiveness of the doctor's services to patients is likely to be significantly reduced or patients are likely to suffer significant inconvenience.
- a GP may seek to be available for less than 26 hours a week, if practising in a partnership. In this case there are two options:
  (i) less than 26 hours but not less than 19 hours
  (ii) less than 19 hours but not less than 13 hours.
- two doctors in partnership may apply for FHSA approval to be jointly available for 26 hours a week.

The NHS Management Executive has issued important guidance to FHSAs on the availability requirements of the 1990 contract.

Strictly speaking, under the Regulations the availability question has to be looked at on the basis of each individual doctor's application in respect of his or her hours and their convenience to patients. The Regulations do not require FHSAs to take partners' availability into account, but nor do they preclude doing so except in circumstances where:

- to do so would result in arrangements which were not convenient to the GP's own patients; or
- the GP whose application is being considered objects.

The Department of Health's view is that, provided these circumstances do not apply, FHSAs may take account of partnership availability. Appeals made against FHSAs' decisions on availability have highlighted several areas where there has been uncertainty about the correct legal interpretation of the availability requirements. The most common instances are summarized below.

- FHSAs **cannot** stipulate which specific days doctors must be available. Under the Regulations it is for doctors to choose which days they wish to be available. The 'convenience to patients' rule then bites on the spread of the hours across the doctor's chosen days. FHSAs may not, for example,

Table 3.7.   List of health-related activities

- activities connected with the organization or training of the medical profession
- activities connected with the provision of medical care or treatment
- activities connected with the improvement of the quality of such care or treatment
- activities connected with the administration of general medical services
- appointments concerning medical education or training
- medical appointments within the health service other than in relation to the provision of general medical services
- medical appointments under the Crown, with government departments or agencies, or public or local authorities
- appointments concerning the regulation of the medical profession or service on the Medical Practices Committee
- membership of a medical audit advisory group

require a doctor to provide a surgery on a Saturday, if that doctor is already available on five other days each week.

- Many FHSAs have agreed local policies as to how they deal with applications by doctors for approval of hours of availability. Nevertheless, each application has to be considered individually against the requirements of the terms of service. FHSAs may not hold that a doctor's proposed hours are inconvenient merely because they do not meet local criteria. There must be a recognized procedure for looking at each doctor's individual circumstances and convenience to patients.
- The Regulations do not specifically require doctors to work the **same** five days every week. There is therefore no bar on doctors working a rota system provided that it meets the 'convenience to patients' test; for example, a fixed and regular rota, which is easily understandable by, and is advertised to, patients.
- FHSAs have the authority, when approving a doctor's hours of availability, to make its approval subject to specified conditions. However, one such condition may **not** be that approval is limited to a certain period (e.g. approving the hours subject to a review in six months). Any conditions laid down must involve an amendment to the proposed hours of availability which, if accepted by the GP, would result in the hours being agreed.
- FHSAs do not have the authority to designate a doctor, who has applied on the basis of full-time availability, as a part-time doctor and to reduce rates of pay accordingly. FHSAs may **only** reduce rates of payment to those appropriate for GPs working part-time, where it is a condition imposed by the MPC that the doctor should work part-time.
- In the case of doctors applying for four-day availability it is not necessary for the 'health-related activities' concerned to be performed on the day for which relief is being sought. Provided these activities are on a fixed and regular basis, a doctor may be entitled to apply for reduced availability on the basis of the cumulative effects of such activities.

Practice area

A doctor may not open premises in an area where, at the time of the application, the MPC considers the number of GPs to be adequate. Subject to this condition, a GP may apply at any time to the FHSA for consent to alter the practice area. (If the FHSA refuses consent, the GP may appeal to the Secretary of State.)

Notification of change of residence

When a GP changes his or her place of residence, the FHSA should be told in writing within 28 days.

Records

A GP should keep adequate records of the illnesses and treatment of patients on forms supplied by the FHSA, and should send these to it on request as soon as possible. Within 14 days of being informed by the FHSA of a patient's death (or not later than one month after otherwise learning of it), a GP should return the records to the FHSA.

Certification

A GP should issue to patients or their personal representatives free of charge the certificates listed in Table 3.8 if they are reasonably required. However, a GP is not obliged to do so if the patient is being attended by another doctor (other than a partner, assistant or deputy) or is not being treated by, or under the supervision of, a doctor. In certain circumstances, a GP may issue a statement, without an examination, advising the patient to refrain from work for a period of up to a month, provided a written report, not more than a month old, has been received from another doctor at a hospital, place of employment or other institution. The other doctor should not be a partner, assistant or deputy.

Accepting fees

A GP must not demand or accept a fee or other remuneration for any treatment, including maternity medical services, whether under the terms of service or not, given to a person for whose treatment he or she is responsible. Doctors must take all practical steps to ensure that any partner, deputy

Table 3.8.   List of prescribed medical certificates

Column 1 *Description of Medical Certificate*	Column 2 *Short title of enactment under or for the purpose of which certificate required*
1. To support a claim to obtain payment either personally or by proxy; to prove inability to work or incapacity for self-support for the purposes of an award by the Secretary of State; or to enable proxy to draw pensions etc.	Naval and Marine Pay and Pensions Act 1865(a) Air Force (Constitution) Act 1917(b) Pensions (Navy, Army, Air Force and Mercantile Marine) Act 1939(c) Personal Injuries (Emergency Provisions) Act 1939(d) Pensions (Mercantile Marine) Act 1942(e) Polish Resettlement Act 1947(f) Home Guard Act 1951(g) Social Security Act 1975(h) Industrial Injuries and Diseases (Old Cases) Act 1975(i) Parts I and III of the Social Security and Housing Benefits Act 1982(j) Parts II and V of, and Schedule 4 to, the Social Security Act 1986(k)
2. To establish pregnancy for the purpose of obtaining welfare foods	Section 13 of the Social Security Act (1988)(l)
3. To establish fitness to receive inhalational analgesia in childbirth	Nurses, Midwives and Health Visitors Act 1979(m)
4. To secure registration of still-birth	Births and Deaths Registration Act 1953(n)
5. To enable payment to be made to an institution or other person in case of mental disorder of persons entitled to payment from public funds	Section 142 of the Mental Health Act 1983(o)
6. To establish unfitness for jury service	Juries Act 1974(p)
7. To establish unfitness to attend for medical examination	National Service Act 1948(q)
8. To support late application for reinstatement in civil employment or notification of non-availability to take up employment, owing to sickness	Reinstatement in Civil Employment Act 1944(r) Reinstatement in Civil Employment Act 1950(s) Reserve Forces Act 1980(t)
9. To enable a person to be registered as an absent voter on grounds of physical incapacity	Representation of the People Act 1983
10. To support application for certificates conferring exemption from charges in respect of drugs, medicines and appliances	National Health Service Act 1977
11. To support a claim by or on behalf of a severely mentally impaired person for exemption from liability to pay the community charge	Local Government Finance Act 1988

continued

Table 3.8. Continued

Column 1 *Description of Medical Certificate*	Column 2 *Short title of enactment under or for the* *purpose of which certificate required*
12. To support a claim by or on behalf of a severely mentally impaired person for exemption from liability to pay the Council Tax or eligibility for a discount in respect of the amount of Council Tax payable	Local Government Finance Act 1992(u)

(a)	28 & 29 Vict. c.73.	(b)	7 & 8 Geo. 5 c.51.
(c)	2 & 3 Geo. 6 c.83.	(d)	2 & 3 Geo. 6 c.82.
(e)	5 & 6 Geo. 6 c.26.	(f)	10 & 11 Geo. 6 c.19.
(g)	15 & 16 Geo. 6 and 1 Eliz. 2 c.8	(h)	1975 c.14.
(i)	1975 c.16.	(j)	1982 c.24.
(k)	1986 c.50.	(l)	1988 c.7.
(m)	1979 c.36.	(n)	1 and 2 Eliz. 2 c.72.
(o)	1983 c.20.	(p)	1974 c.23.
(q)	11 & 12 Geo. 6 c.64.	(r)	7 & 8 Geo. 6 c.15.
(s)	14 & 15 Geo. 6 c.10.	(t)	1980 c.9.
(u)	1992 c.14.		

or assistant does not demand or accept any remuneration for treatment given to their patients unless, of course, the partner, deputy or assistant would have been entitled to charge if the patient had been on his or her own list.

There are, however, certain specific circumstances in which a GP may accept a fee. These are listed in Table 3.9.

There are other certificates and reports which are not part of a GP's NHS obligations to patients. The fee for these is a matter to be agreed between the GP and the patient. The BMA issues agreed and recommended lists of fees for these procedures.

A doctor must not demand or accept a fee or other remuneration from a patient for prescribing or supplying any drug or chemical reagent or appliance, unless the patient requires a medicine solely in anticipation of the onset of an ailment outside the United Kingdom but for which he or she is not requiring treatment when the medicine is prescribed or supplied.

Prescribing and dispensing

A GP is required to supply drugs or listed appliances needed for a patient's immediate treatment before a supply can be obtained elsewhere. In the course of treating a patient under general medical services, a GP must not issue a prescription for a drug or other substance listed in schedule 10 to the

Table 3.9.   Specific circumstances in which a GP may accept a fee

(a)   from any statutory body for services rendered for the purpose of that body's statutory functions

(b)   from any body, employer or school for a routine medical examination of persons for whose welfare the body, employer or school is responsible, or an examination of such persons for the purpose of advising the body, employer or school of any administrative action they might take

(c)   for treatment which is not of a type usually provided by general practitioners and which is given:

  (i)   pursuant to the provisions of section 65 of the Act, or
  (ii) in a registered nursing home which is not providing services under the Act

  if, in either case, the doctor is serving on the staff of a hospital providing services under the Act as a specialist providing treatment of the kind the patient requires and if, within 7 days of giving the treatment, the doctor supplies the FHSA, on a form provided by it for the purpose, with such information about the treatment as it may require

(d)   under Section 158 of the Road Traffic Act 1988(a)

(e)   from a dentist in respect of the provision at his request of an anaesthetic for a person for whom the dentist is providing general dental services

(f)   when he treats a patient under paragraph 4(3), in which case he shall be entitled to demand and accept a reasonable fee (recoverable under paragraph 39) for any treatment given, if he gives the patient a receipt on a form suplied by the FHSA

(g)   for attending and examining (but not otherwise treating) a patient at his request at a police station in connection with proceedings which the police are minded to bring against him

(h)   for treatment consisting of an immunization for which no remuneration is payable by the FHSA in pursuance of the Statement made under regulation 34 and which is requested in connection with travel abroad

(i)   for circumcising a patient for whom such an operation is requested on religious grounds and is not needed on any medical ground

(j)   for prescribing or providing drugs which a patient requires to have in his possession solely in anticipation of the onset of an ailment while he is outside the United Kingdom but for which he is not requiring treatment when the medicine is prescribed

(k)   for a medical examination to enable a decision to be made whether or not it is inadvisable on medical grounds for a person to wear a seat belt

(l)   where the person is not one to whom any of paragraphs (a), (b) or (c) of section 38(1) of the Act(b) applies (including by reason of regulations under section 38(6) of that Act), for testing the sight of that person

(m)   where he is a doctor who is authorized or required by an FHSA under regulation 20 of the Pharmaceutical Regulations to provide drugs, medicines or appliances to a patient and provides for that patient, otherwise than under pharmaceutical services, any Scheduled drug.

(a) 1988 c.53.
(b) 1977 c.49 section 38 was amended by the Health and Social Security Act 1984 (c.48), section 1(3), by S.I. 1985/39, article 7(11), and by the Health and Medicines Act 1988 (c.49), section 13(1).

Regulations (the 'black list') for supply under the NHS. In the case of a drug listed under schedule 11, a doctor may prescribe only in certain circumstances. A GP may prescribe these items privately, but may not charge for doing so. The GP can only charge for the item itself if he or she is already entitled to dispense to a patient and the GP can only do so for a particular course of treatment.

Practice leaflets

A GP or partnership should prepare a practice leaflet including the information in Table 3.10 on page 28.

The leaflet should be reviewed at least annually to maintain accuracy and an up-to-date copy should be available to the FHSA, each patient on the doctor's list and anyone who reasonably requires one.

Inquiries about prescriptions and referrals

The GP should be prepared to answer any inquiries from the FHSA relating to:

- any prescriptions issued
- referrals to other NHS services.

Annual reports

A GP or partnership should provide the FHSA annually with a report containing the information in Table 3.11. The information in paragraph 3 of the table need only be supplied if the FHSA requests it, having considered whether the information is available from another source and having consulted the LMC. The information in paragraph 4 of the table need only be supplied if the FHSA requests it and the GP is not supplying the information already in order to qualify for health promotion or disease management payments. Each report should be compiled for a 12 month period ending 31 March and should be sent to the FHSA by 30 June.

Conclusion

This commentary is selective, not comprehensive. Not all of the paragraphs in the terms of service have been covered and only a brief summary of those referred to has been provided. If any problem arises, a GP should refer to the Regulations and if necessary seek the advice and assistance of the LMC secretary or BMA regional office.

Table 3.10. Information to be included in practice leaflets

Personal and professional details of the doctor:

1 full name
2 sex
3 medical qualifications registered by the General Medical Council
4 date and place of first registration as medical practitioner

Practice information:

5 the times approved by the FHSA during which the doctor is personally available for consultation by his patients at his practice premises
6 whether an appointments system is operated by the doctor for consultations at his practice premises
7 if there is an appointments system, the method of obtaining a non-urgent appointment and the method of obtaining an urgent appointment
8 the method of obtaining a non-urgent domiciliary visit and the method of obtaining an urgent domiciliary visit
9 the doctor's arrangements for providing personal medical services when he is not personally available
10 the method by which patients are to obtain repeat prescriptions from the doctor
11 if the doctor's practice is a dispensing practice, the arrangements for dispensing prescriptions
12 if the doctor provides clinics for his patients, their frequency, duration and purpose
13 the numbers of staff, other than doctors, assisting the doctor in his practice, and a description of their roles
14 whether the doctor provides maternity medical services, contraceptive services, child health surveillance services, minor surgery services
15 whether the doctor works single-handed, in partnership, part-time or on a job sharing basis, or within a group practice
16 the nature of any arrangements whereby the doctor or his staff receive patients' comments on his provision of general medical services
17 the geographical boundary of his practice area by reference to a sketch, diagram or plan
18 whether the doctor's practice premises have suitable access for all disabled patients and, if not, the reasons why they are unsuitable for particular types of disability
19 if an assistant is employed, details for him as specified in paragraphs 1–5 of this table
20 if the practice either is a general practitioner training practice for the purposes of the National Health Service (Vocational Training) Regulations 1979 or undertakes the teaching of undergraduate medical students, the nature of arrangements for drawing this to the attention of patients.

Table 3.11. Information to be provided in annual reports

1 Particulars of the doctor's other commitments as a medical practitioner, including:

  (a) a description of any posts held, and
  (b) a description of all work undertaken

  and including, in each case, the annual hourly commitment, except that where a doctor has notified the FHSA of such other commitments in a previous annual report, the report need only contain information relating to any changes in those commitments.

2 As respects orders for drugs and appliances, the doctor's arrangements for the issue of repeat prescriptions to patients.

3 Information relating to the referral of patients to other services under the Act during the period of the report:

  (a) as respects those by the doctor to specialists:

    (i) the total number of patients referred as in-patients
    (ii) the total number of patients referred as out-patients

    by reference in each case to which clinical specialty applies, and specifying in each case the name of the hospital concerned; and

  (b) the total number of cases of which the doctor is aware (by reference to the clinical specialty) in which a patient referred himself to services under the Act.

4 Information relating to the numbers of patients on the doctor's list:

  (a) who are diabetic
  (b) who are asthmatic and
  (c) to whom the doctor has given advice, in accordance with paragraph 12(2) of schedule 2, about:

    (i)   the patient's weight
    (ii) the use of tobacco, or
    (iii) the consumption of alcohol.

4 The basic practice allowance

Principals and assistants

Is the contractual status of a salaried partner the same as that of a salaried assistant? What is the difference between a principal and an associate? Many GPs cannot answer these questions correctly, yet ignorance of their own status and that of their colleagues can expose them to considerable risk.

Some definitions are provided in the Red Book and FHSAs use these to decide which payments a doctor is eligible to receive. The most important distinction is between principals and other doctors working in NHS general practice who are not principals.

A *principal* is defined as a practitioner in contract with an FHSA, as either a single-handed practitioner (whether or not within a group) or a partner in a partnership. Under the contract, every principal accepts those responsibilities defined in the terms of service, including being responsible for any doctor or practice staff he or she employs. A principal is eligible for most of the payments specified in the Red Book, is self-employed and (if in a partnership) participates in partnership decisions and is free to accept patients onto his or her list.

The main types of GP principal are listed in Box 4.1.

Box 4.1: Types of GP principals

- full-time practitioner: unrestricted principal providing general medical services for at least 26 hours a week
- three-quarter time practitioner: unrestricted principal providing general medical services for at least 19 hours a week
- half-time practitioner: unrestricted principal providing general medical services for at least 13 hours a week
- job sharer: unrestricted principal who provides general medical services for at least 26 hours a week jointly with another unrestricted principal

---

A *salaried partner* is a partner who draws a share of the profits in the form of a salary. This arrangement may be challenged by the FHSA if it insists that all partners must have a share of partnership profits calculated as a fraction or a percentage of the total profits, rather than as a salary.

Unless a principal works single-handed (whether or not within a group) the FHSA must be satisfied that he or she is truly a partner. NHS Regulations state that to be recognized as a partner, a full-time practitioner must receive a share of the partnership profits which is at least one-third of the share enjoyed by the partner with the largest share. This means that in a two doctor partnership the maximum ratio between the shares of the senior and junior partners is three to one, with the junior partner receiving a quarter of the profits.

The Regulations also state that a three-quarter time partner must receive a share of the profits which is at least one-quarter of the profits enjoyed by the partner with the greatest share, and a half-time practitioner at least one-fifth of the greatest share.

Doctors who are not principals

The following are not recognized as principals; they do not have a contract with the FHSA and are not eligible to claim payments from the FHSA (apart from certain specific reimbursements).

Associate: practitioner employed by an isolated single-handed practitioner or job sharers in conjunction with another single-handed isolated practitioner or practitioners, with the agreement of the FHSA or Health Board.

Assistant: practitioner either employed by a principal with the consent of the FHSA or working within a partnership but not as a partner.

Trainee practitioner: fully registered practitioner training in general practice and employed by an approved trainer. (Trainers and trainees can claim payments from the FHSA relating to the traineeship.)

Locum: doctor employed by a practitioner to assist on a temporary or occasional basis.

It is vital that a practitioner is certain about his or her status before accepting an appointment in general practice.

Box 4.2: Rights and responsibilities of principals

- principals have a contract with an FHSA and receive a wide range of payments described in the Red Book
- principals in a partnership must receive certain minimum shares of the profits
- principals are responsible for the acts and omissions of doctors they employ, e.g. associates, assistants, trainees and locums

Basic practice allowance

The Basic Practice Allowance (BPA) is the key element of a GP's income for providing NHS general medical services. Other allowances depend on entitlement to the BPA. Doctors should establish their entitlement to a full or partial BPA before applying to join an FHSA list. No BPA will be paid to a doctor working within a partnership who is not deemed to be a partner. The BPA is a payment which recognizes the continuing responsibility and basic costs involved in providing general medical services during the normal working week, and reflects those standing expenses or overheads (apart from premises and staff) which do not vary proportionately with list size.

Under the 1990 contract the conditions for paying the BPA have changed significantly. Eligibility now relates almost solely to list size and there is no requirement to devote a substantial amount of time to general practice (the former so called '20 hour rule'). Requirements in respect of availability are now included in the terms of service (e.g. the requirement that a full time GP should be available for at least 26 hours a week).

Full-time practitioners are eligible for a full BPA if they provide general medical services and have 1200 or more patients on their personal lists, or are in a partnership with an average list of at least 1200 patients. (Under the old contract the list size requirement for payment of full BPA was 1000 patients.)

Practitioners will be eligible for a lower rate BPA if they have at least 400 but no more than 1199 patients on their personal lists, or are in a partnership with an average list within this range. Payment will be a lump sum for the first 400 patients plus additional amounts at different rates for each patient up to 600, 800, 1000 and 1200 patients.

Job sharers

Job sharers are jointly eligible for a single BPA at the appropriate rate, according to their combined list size (irrespective of personal list sizes) or the average list size if they are members of a partnership.

Part-time practitioners

A part-time practitioner will be eligible for only one BPA. A half-time practitioner may not earn a level of BPA greater than that payable for a list of 600 patients, and no three-quarter time practitioner may earn a BPA greater than that for a list of 900 patients.

Calculating partnership average list size

To calculate a partnership's average list size the FHSA adds together the personal list sizes of all partners and divides the total by a divisor which takes into account any fractions worked by part-timers. Each partner is then credited with the average number of patients multiplied by the appropriate figure reflecting the partner's time commitment, subject to the limits on BPA for part-time practitioners specified above. For example, in a partnership of three full-time GPs and one half-time GP, the divisor will be 7 (7 × 0.50 = 3 + 0.50), while in a partnership of two full-time GPs, one three-quarter time GP and one half-time GP, the divisor will be 13 (13 × 0.25 = 2 + 0.75 + 0.50).

Box 4.3: Full BPA: to be eligible practitioners must:

- provide general medical services
- have at least 1200 patients on their personal list or be in a partnership with this average list size

---

Leave payment

Part of the BPA expected to be paid during a financial year can be taken in advance as a 'leave payment' for a holiday or period of study leave of at least one week; leave payment should be applied for by 15 April in the financial year when leave is to be taken. Leave payments are useful in improving a practice's cash flow.

The total amount drawn cannot exceed one-fifth of the BPA and is recovered through quarterly deductions. Thus, a leave payment taken in May must be applied for by 15 April and will be fully recovered by the following 31 March.

Box 4.4: Leave payment

- this is a part-payment of the BPA in advance
- applications must be made 15 April
- total leave payment cannot exceed one-fifth of the BPA

GPs only qualify for the following allowances if they are receiving the BPA:

- designated area allowance
- seniority allowance
- assistant allowance.

The full amount of these allowances is only paid to a GP receiving the full BPA. The actual amount paid to a GP who is not eligible for a full BPA is calculated as follows:

$$\frac{\text{amount of BPA received}}{\text{maximum rate of BPA}} \times \text{allowance}$$

The group practice allowance (a special incentive to encourage group practice) and the vocational training allowance were abolished when the 1990 contract was introduced.

Allowance for practising in a designated area

Designated areas are areas defined as under-doctored by the Medical Practices Committee; currently there are none and no new payments are made for this purpose. However, a very small and declining number of GPs may still be receiving payments for practising in areas previously classified as designated.

Payment of a Type 1 Allowance was made to GPs whose main surgery was in a locality that had been designated as under-doctored for at least three years. Payment was made whilst the area remained designated or for a concessionary period of a further three years after this designation ceased. A Type 2 Allowance was paid to doctors whose main surgery was in an area continuously designated as under-doctored for one year with average lists of over 3000 patients. The payment continued for a two year concessionary period after the average list size fell below 3000.

Because average list sizes have dropped and designated areas have disappeared, any GP still receiving this allowance is now in the concessionary payment period.

Seniority allowance

This allowance is paid to any GP who has both completed a specified number of years since registration with the General Medical Council (GMC) and a specified length of service as an NHS GP. The three levels of seniority allowance are related to the length of registration and service (*see* Box 5.1).

Box 5.1: Three levels of seniority allowance

first: registered with GMC for 11 years or more
          principal GP for at least 7 years
second: registered with GMC for 18 years or more
          principal GP for at least 14 years
third: registered with GMC for 25 years or more
          principal GP for at least 21 years

If the qualifying conditions are met and the GP is receiving a full BPA, the full seniority allowance will be paid. Pro rata payments are made to GPs receiving partial BPA. Job sharers are assessed for seniority payments on an individual basis and these are reduced pro rata according to the doctor's hours of availability.

The rules outlined in Boxes 5.2 and 5.3 describe how to work out both length of registration and service as an NHS principal.

Box 5.2: Calculating length of registration

- registration by the GMC (or by the Medical Registration Council of the Republic of Ireland) counts from the date of provisional (but not temporary or limited) registration, or otherwise the date of full registration
- the FHSA may allow a GP to count registration from the date of first registration by an overseas authority if the qualification is recognized by the GMC for provisional, full, temporary or limited registration
- registration must normally be continuous; any break may affect a GP's entitlement to seniority payments

---

Box 5.3: Calculating length of service as an NHS GP principal

- all service as an unrestricted NHS GP since 1948, ignoring absences due to national service, holidays, sick leave, study leave or a hospital attachment if a GP's name remained on the medical list
- if a GP resigns from the medical list but returns after more than six months, there is a qualifying period before the GP is entitled to a seniority payment. This varies according to the length of the break; between six and 18 months requires a qualifying period of six months, while a break of more than 90 months requires a qualifying period of 48 months. Service as an assistant, locum or principal during a break may be taken into account. Service in HM Forces in a recognized post is not regarded as a break. Service under Regulation 19(9) and 19(6)(temporary arrangements for conducting a practice) is taken into account
- claims for recognition of service as a medical officer in HM Forces or certain posts in diplomatic missions abroad should be made to the FHSA

Allowance for employing an assistant

An allowance for employing a *full-time assistant* is paid to:

- a single-handed full-time GP (or two job sharers) with a list of at least 3000 patients
- a partnership of full-time GPs (including job sharers) with a minimum combined list of 3000 patients for the first full-time GP (or pair of job sharers) plus an average of 2500 patients for each other full-time GP (or pair of job sharers)
- a partnership of at least one full-time GP (or two job sharers) plus one or more part-time GPs with a minimum combined list of 3000 patients for the first full-time GP (or two job sharers), 2500 patients for each other full-time GP (or two job sharers), 1875 patients for each three-quarter-time GP and 1250 patients for each half-time GP.

If the assistant is employed part-time on NHS general medical services the full allowance will be reduced.

An addition of half the appropriate rate will be paid for employing *an assistant working half-time or more* to:

- a single-handed full-time GP (or two job sharers) with a list of at least 2500 patients

- a partnership of full-time GPs (including job sharers), with a minimum combined list of 2500 patients for the first full-time practitioner (or two job sharers) plus an average of 2250 patients for each other full-time practitioner (or two job sharers)
- a partnership of at least one full-time GP (or two job sharers) plus one or more part-time GPs with a minimum combined list of 2500 patients for the first full-time GP (or set of two job sharers), 2250 for each other full-time GP (or job sharers), 1687 for each three-quarter-time GP and 1125 for each half-time GP.

The allowance is reduced if the assistant is employed less than half-time on NHS general medical services.

The list size requirements for a half-time assistant's allowance are relaxed for single-handed doctors, job sharers and partnerships receiving substantial rural practice payments.

Box 5.4: The assistant's allowance

- single-handed practitioners, job sharers and partnerships are eligible, depending on list size
- list size requirement is reduced if half-time allowance is claimed
- list size requirement is also reduced if the practice is receiving substantial rural practice payments and is claiming only a half-time assistant's allowance

---

Eligibility for this allowance depends on partnership average list size, not individual list size. Only one allowance can be paid for each assistant employed.

All list size requirements are subject to a tolerance of 100 for full-time, 75 for three-quarter-time and 50 for half-time practitioners. Those who qualify initially for the allowance will not lose it until the beginning of the quarter after the list has fallen by at least the amount of the tolerance below the lower list size limit.

Claims for an assistant's allowance should be made on form FP80.

There are very few assistants employed in general practice for whom this allowance is claimed, because its size is small in comparison with the allowances paid for a partner.

☐6 The associate allowance

THIS allowance enables single-handed GPs in isolated areas jointly to employ an associate doctor so that they can have time off for leisure and training, in circumstances where continuous duty would otherwise be an intrinsic feature of general medical services.

Associates should normally work in a single locality. In most cases one associate doctor will be employed jointly between two adjacent practices, although the FHSA or Health Board may agree to an associate being employed between three practitioners.

An associate must undertake the normal range of general medical services provided by the employing principal, who remains responsible under the terms of service for the associate's acts and omissions.

GPs employing assistants are not eligible for this scheme.

In fact, very few GPs in England can qualify for this allowance.

The eligibility criteria are listed in Box 6.1.

Box 6.1: Eligibility for the associate allowance

A single-handed GP (or job sharer) must be:
- receiving rural practice payments, or
- sole practitioner(s) on an island, **and**
- receiving an inducement payment, or
- in a practice more than 10 miles from the nearest practitioner's main surgery or nearest district general hospital

---

Associate doctor

The associate must satisfy all of these conditions:

- meet the requirements of the NHS (Vocational Training) Regulations 1979
- not be on any FHSA or Health Board medical list whilst an associate
- have a full-time commitment to general medical services duties between the two or more employing practitioners
- be under 70.

Applying for approval

Application for approval of the employment of an associate and claims for the allowance are made on form FP/AA. A copy of the associate's contract of employment and details of arrangements for sharing the associate's time between the employing GPs must be provided. The form will ask which employing GP is responsible for administering the associate's contract and should be paid the allowance.

Employing an associate normally disbars those GPs receiving inducement payments from claiming reimbursement of locum fees and expenses.

The employing practitioner is responsible for paying the associate and deducting NI and income tax. An associate may join the NHS superannuation scheme.

The employing practitioners may decide what rate of pay to give the associate, but the FHSA or Health Board pays an allowance as specified in Schedule 1 to the Red Book which allows for incremental progression. It also reimburses an allowance for the associate's use of a car.

An associate may claim various expenses, including removal expenses, directly from the FHSA or Health Board.

The Red Book specifies that two-thirds of an associate's subscription to a professional defence organization will be reimbursed and provides for payment of the postgraduate education allowance. It also describes how the schemes for additional payments during confinement or sickness apply to both the associate and employing practitioners.

7 Absences from practice

Additional payments for sickness

GPs away from the practice because of illness receive normal remuneration and may receive an additional allowance to pay for a locum or deputy, depending on list size. This allowance may not cover the full cost of the locum, and the GP will have to pay the rest. The scheme applies to GPs receiving the BPA and providing unrestricted general medical services. Payments for sickness will be reduced pro rata if less than a full BPA is paid.

Practitioners receiving an associate allowance may qualify for help with the cost of employing a locum during an associate's sickness absence.

Level of payment

Payments vary according to length of service in the NHS (*see* Box 7.1).

Box 7.1: Level of payments during sickness

length of service	*scale of payment*
less than 1 year	1 month's full payment and, after 4 months' service, 2 months' half payment
during second year	2 months' full and 2 months' half payment
during third year	4 months' full and 4 months' half payment
during fourth and fifth years	5 months' full and 5 months' half payment
after 5 years' service	6 months' full and 6 months' half payment

---

The payment is calculated by deducting from the period of benefit appropriate to the doctor's service on the first day of absence, the total period for which payment has already been made during the preceding 12 months. The meaning of the term 'service' is defined in the Red Book.

Conditions for payment

Payments are only made if one or more locums or deputies from outside the practice are employed. It is accepted that a single-handed GP will normally need to engage a locum or deputy when incapacitated. However, an assistant employed by a single-handed GP will be expected to cover the practice unaided for up to four weeks if the list is 2700 or less. Doctors in partnerships or groups will be expected to provide cross cover as far as possible and additional payments will be made only if a GP's absence leaves the other doctors with a high average number of patients to care for (*see* Box 7.2).

Box 7.2: Average number of patients per remaining partner needed to qualify for additional payments during sickness

Duration/ expected duration of incapacity	*Average number of patients*		
	Full-time GP	Three-quarter-time GP	Half-time GP
not more than two weeks	3600 or more	2700 or more	1800 or more
not more than six weeks	3100 or more	2325 or more	1550 or more
more than six weeks	2700 or more	2025 or more	1350 or more

When calculating the average number of patients, an FHSA assumes each part-time GP has on his or her personal list the number of patients set out above. Once these figures have been deducted from the total partnership or group list, the balance will be averaged between the remaining GPs. If a partnership or group employs a full-time assistant (or equivalent part-time assistants) other than a trainee practitioner, the assistant will be deemed to care for up to 2700 patients and this number will therefore be deducted from the total number of patients on the lists of the partners or group members before calculating the average number of patients to be cared for by the remaining partners or group members. Similarly, if a partnership or group employs a part-time assistant, the assistant will be deemed to be able to care for that proportion of 2700 patients corresponding to the proportion of a full-time commitment the assistant works.

The FHSA, after consulting the LMC, may waive these requirements if the practice covers a large geographical area, or the GPs' ages or health restrict their capacity to take on the additional workload, or the prevalence of sickness in the practice area is unusually high.

No payments are made if the period of incapacity is less than a week or if a GP is absent because of an accident which allows financial compensation to be recovered.

For payments to be made under the scheme medical certificates need to be submitted to the FHSA, and if requested a GP must agree to be examined by a doctor nominated by the FHSA.

Box 7.3: Additional payments for sickness

- the payments contribute towards the cost of a locum or deputy from outside the practice
- eligibility depends on length of absence and practice list size
- duration of payment depends on length of service

Basis of payment

A full-time GP eligible for full payment and employing a full-time locum or deputy (working 'normal' hours on at least five days a week, or the equivalent spread over six days) from outside the practice, will be reimbursed the actual amount paid or the maximum allowance, whichever is less.

A part-time GP will receive a reduced reimbursement: either half or three-quarters of maximum, depending on hours of availability. Payments are also reduced if the locum is employed less than full-time.

Payment varies according to a different formula if the deputy is a principal on an FHSA list. Although the same overall limit applies, payment is calculated at a maximum rate of three-quarters of the standard capitation fees earned by the sick GP. More than one locum or deputy may be employed, but total reimbursement will not exceed that paid for one full-time equivalent. These reimbursements may be abated if a GP's private practice income exceeds 10% of his or her total practice income.

Assistants

If a GP employs an assistant for whom an allowance is paid, additional payments during sickness may be paid if the assistant falls ill.

Additional payments during confinement

A similar scheme to that for sickness payments applies to women GPs who are absent owing to pregnancy and childbirth. The payments supplement normal remuneration and are paid if a GP remains on the medical list and intends to continue in general practice, and only if a locum or deputy from outside the practice is employed. All women GPs providing unrestricted general medical services and in receipt of a BPA are eligible. A part-time GP can claim half or three-quarters of the allowance, depending on her availability.

Duration of payment

Payment is for a maximum of 13 weeks, even though a GP may be away for a longer period. A doctor who is absent because of illness before or after the 13 week period covered by this scheme may claim additional payments for sickness.

The GP must state that she intends to return to general practice within a reasonable period after the birth.

Box 7.4: Additional payments during confinement

- eligibility is not related to list size
- payments are made for up to 13 weeks
- the applicant must declare her intention to return to general practice after the birth

---

How to claim

Claims should be made early in pregnancy and must be accompanied by a certificate of expected confinement or a similar private certificate.

Absence of assistants

A doctor receiving an assistant's allowance may claim payments for employing outside help during the assistant's confinement.

Locum allowance for rural single-handed practitioners attending educational courses

A single-handed doctor receiving rural practice payments and absent from the practice on an accredited postgraduate educational course may receive a special payment (in addition to normal remuneration) towards the cost of a locum or other deputy doctor looking after the practice.

The scheme applies to single-handed doctors receiving rural practice payments (except those with an associate allowance, who are expected to arrange for their associate doctor to look after the practice during their absence). The course must last at least a full day. This allowance is only paid if a locum is actually employed and may cover both the course and associated travelling time.

If a doctor already employs an assistant, the assistant will be expected to look after the practice unaided for up to four weeks, if the list size is no more than 2700.

Basis of payment

If a locum who is not a principal on an FHSA list is engaged, payments the employing doctor has made to the locum will be reimbursed up to the weekly maximum stated in the Red Book. If the doctor is absent for less than one week, locum payments will be reimbursed at up to one fifth of the weekly rate for every full day for which the locum was engaged, up to the weekly maximum.

If the locum is on an FHSA medical list and has his or her own practice, payment will be subject to a maximum rate representing three quarters of the standard capitation fees (including the higher rates for elderly patients) due to the absent GP.

If a GP engages more than one locum, the total figure reimbursed cannot exceed that payable for a single locum. If one locum is on a medical list and the other is not, the respective reimbursements will be calculated as stated above.

Payments will not be abated if the gross income from private practice undertaken by the doctor is less than 10% of total practice income. If gross receipts from private practice are greater, payments will be abated by 10% if between 10% and 20% of gross income is from private practice, by 20% if between 20% and 30% is, and so on. However, if a locum does not cover for any private work or is not qualified to do so and the FHSA accepts this position, it excludes from the calculation any income from work which the locum does not undertake for the absent doctor.

It is important to ensure that expenses incurred when employing a locum are shown gross in the practice accounts and that payments from the FHSA are shown as income, in the same way as capitation fees and other receipts.

Claims for payment

The doctor's responsible FHSA makes the payment and provides application and claim forms. A GP should apply to the FHSA as soon as a locum has been arranged so that the FHSA can decide as soon as possible whether the application is acceptable.

Claims for payment should be submitted when practice is resumed or when the locum's employment ends, whichever is the earlier. The certificate on the reverse side of the form must be completed and signed by each locum for whom payment is claimed.

If there is a change in locum arrangements, the FHSA must be told immediately, and no further claims should be submitted until the change is accepted.

Allowances for prolonged study leave

This allowance, which provides financial support to a GP who takes prolonged study leave in the interests of medicine or the NHS, is rarely claimed. Prolonged study differs in scope and depth from a refresher course and should be capable of significantly extending a GP's professional or administrative skills and knowledge. Study leave solely for the purpose of obtaining a higher professional qualification is not normally eligible. Advice about the scheme can be obtained from the regional adviser in general practice or the FHSA.

Key features of the scheme are:

- absence should normally last between 10 weeks and 12 months
- payments are in the form of an educational allowance and (where applicable) a contribution towards the cost of employing a locum or deputy from outside the practice
- the locum allowance is calculated in a similar way to that paid during sickness, except that there are no list size criteria
- the application should be sent to the regional postgraduate dean who forwards it, together with the views of the regional postgraduate committee, to the Secretary of State who decides whether the proposal is acceptable.

Box 7.5: Allowance for prolonged study leave

- absence normally lasts between 10 weeks and 12 months
- payments take the form of an educational allowance and (where appropriate) a locum allowance
- eligibility for a locum allowance is unrelated to list size
- applications, submitted via the regional postgraduate dean, are determined by the Secretary of State

---

Temporary arrangements for carrying on a practice

The NHS (General Medical Services) Regulations provide for the temporary care of patients, if their GP has ceased to be included in the medical list, or has been suspended from the medical register, or is not carrying out his or her terms-of-service obligations adequately. The arrangements for payments to the GP appointed to care for these patients under Regulation 25(2) or 25(6) are explained in paragraph 78 of the Red Book.

8 Capitation fees and calculating list size

STANDARD capitation fees are paid at three rates according to the patient's age on the last day of the preceding quarter:

- under 65 years
- 65 to 74 years
- 75 years and over.

Fees are paid quarterly at one quarter of the annual rate. (Capitation fees for child health surveillance and deprivation are also paid quarterly at one quarter of the annual rate.)

The calculation of lists is described in paragraph 73 of the Red Book. Under the 1990 contract patients' ages are calculated quarterly, not annually as previously. As soon as possible after the beginning of each quarter, the FHSA will notify the GP of:

- the number of patients on the list in each of the three age groups
- the number of children for whom he or she has agreed to provide child health surveillance
- the number of patients for whom a deprivation payment is due, in each group, and the level of fee they attract
- the number of patients for whom a rural practice payment is due.

If the FHSA is told of a patient's acceptance onto a GP's list within 48 hours of the start of a quarter, and it is satisfied that the patient was accepted on or before the first day of the quarter, the patient will be included in the count of patients on the first day of the quarter. Every GP should send acceptances to the FHSA as soon as possible. This helps the FHSA to spread its workload, to increase the accuracy of the count at the start of the quarter, and to speed up transfer of medical records between practices.

How to challenge an FHSA's estimate of list size

A GP wishing to challenge the FHSA's count of patients must tell the FHSA of his or her intention within 10 days of being notified of the numbers on his or her list. Objections cannot be made after this 10 day period. Having given notice of a challenge, the GP should submit to the FHSA, within 21 days of receiving the original notification, any evidence reasonably required to settle the dispute.

Box 8.1: Challenging the FHSA's estimate of list size

- notice of challenge must be submitted within 10 days of receiving notification of list size
- the onus is on the GP to submit evidence to challenge the FHSA's figures, within 21 days of being notified of list size

9 Deprivation payments

A doctor providing general medical services to a patient residing in an area identified as deprived, will be eligible to receive a deprivation payment for that patient. Deprived areas are determined by the Secretary of State following consultation with the profession, and are based on the Jarman Index.

The FHSA will pay the appropriate fee on the first day of each quarter for each patient who attracts a deprivation payment. There are three levels of payment, according to the extent of deprivation in the area where the patient lives.

10 Initial practice allowances and inducement payments

Initial practice allowances

Initial practice allowances (IPAs) support practices which are essential to meet patients' needs but are not otherwise viable. There are two types of allowance.

Type one allowance: single-handed practices in designated areas

This is available to full-time and job sharing practitioners setting up a new single-handed practice, or filling a vacancy in a small single-handed practice, in a designated medical practice area.

A 'small single-handed' practice is one in which the total annual income from capitation fees (including deprivation payments), child health surveillance fees and basic practice allowance, calculated on the size of the list at the date of succeeding to the vacancy, could fall short of the allowance in the first year.

Who is eligible?

To qualify for the allowance a GP must have been:

- in general practice for not less than one year as a principal, assistant, associate or trainee, or
- fully registered for not less than three years.

How it is paid

The allowance is paid for up to four years to guarantee the practice a minimum income, according to the scale detailed in the Red Book. If the GP is setting up a new practice, the full allowance is paid in the first year. If the practitioner is succeeding to an established practice, he or she receives the allowance less the income which the practice attracts from capitation fees, deprivation payments, child health surveillance fees and basic practice allowance (excluding additions) that are payable in respect of the patients transferred to the incoming practitioner. In subsequent years there is no differentiation between the payments to GPs who have set up a new practice and those who have succeeded to an existing practice: the allowance is paid minus the income the practice attracts from capitation fees etc.

There are currently no designated areas in England and Wales and therefore no new type one initial practice allowances can be paid.

Type two: practices in special areas

This allowance is paid in areas selected by the Health Department in consultation with the MPC, taking account of reports from FHSAs, which will have consulted LMCs. Type two allowances are appropriate for areas of housing development where a rapid and considerable population increase is expected and it is desirable from the outset for experienced GPs to establish a practice and primary care team working with other local health services. The first and second GPs must be full time, as must a majority of the GPs.

The allowance provides a guaranteed net income at flat rates for both the first and second practitioner in a practice recognized as attracting a type two allowance. It will be payable for up to five years from the date the first GP takes up his or her appointment.

Appointing a GP

The first GP will be appointed by the Medical Practices Committee after advertising the post; he or she will normally have been qualified for 10 years, have spent two years in hospital posts and five years in a busy general practice in the UK.

The second GP will normally be appointed as a partner to the first GP and the usual arrangements for filling a partnership vacancy apply.

Full details of the scheme are given in paragraphs 41.12 to 41.21 of the Red Book.

Initial practice allowances: preserved rights

Doctors who at 31 March 1990 were eligible for a Type C Initial Practice Allowance under the provisions of paragraph 40 of the Red Book in force at that time will continue to receive the allowance as long as they remain on an FHSA medical list and satisfy the qualifying conditions.

The amounts for the four years of a Type C allowance are shown in the schedule attached to paragraph 81 of the new Red Book.

Inducement payments

Eligibility and payment

An inducement payment will be available for full-time or job sharing GPs practising in an area where the FHSA (after consultation with the Medical

Practices Committee) recognizes that it is essential to maintain a medical practice, although the area may be sparsely populated or in some way unattractive to GPs. Very few inducement payments are available in England and Wales.

A practitioner who wishes to be considered should contact the FHSA; eligibility and any sum payable are decided by the Secretary of State on the merits of each case and are reviewed annually.

Seniority allowance, associate allowance and sickness payments

For the purposes of seniority allowance, associate allowance and sickness payments a doctor who receives an inducement payment will be treated as if he or she has a list of at least 1200 patients.

11 Rural practice payments scheme

THIS scheme provides for mileage payments to be made from a central fund which is fixed annually and known as the Rural Practice Fund. The total amount available is divided by the number of units credited to GPs throughout England and Wales, and the payment to each individual GP is calculated by multiplying the number of units to which the GP is entitled by the value of each unit. The scheme was radically revised on 1 April 1991; effectively a mileage scheme has replaced the rural practice payments scheme in that payments are no longer restricted to GPs with patients in rural areas.

Who is eligible?

A single-handed GP or partnership may be paid rural practice units if at least 20% of the patients live at least three miles from the main surgery by the normal route. If the proportion of patients falls below 20%, the GP or partnership ceases to be eligible, except that if the drop is not below 19%, the FHSA may continue payments for not more than four successive quarters.

How is the main surgery defined?

Calculations are based on the distance from the main surgery; if a practice has several surgeries and there is doubt about which is the main surgery, FHSAs will determine the premises from which the units are calculated, in consultation with LMCs. This decision will take account of surgery times, the number of patients seen in each location, and comments from the doctors. If there are substantial changes in the practice, the surgery from which payments are calculated may be altered, but before doing so the FHSA will consult the LMC and the practice. A doctor in group practice or partnership will have his or her units calculated from the group or partnership's main surgery unless he or she spends less than half his or her total surgery time there, in which case another surgery may be used for the calculations.

How to calculate units

A GP will be credited with the appropriate number of units calculated on the first day of each quarter. Reinstatements or removals from lists relating to the previous quarter received after the second day but within the first month of the new quarter will be taken into account retrospectively.

Each patient who qualifies will attract units on the following grounds, except that no patient may attract units for both blocked route and residence in a special district.

- distance
- walking
- blocked route
- residence in a special district.

Units for distance and walking will only be credited for patients who live not less than three miles from the main surgery by the normal route.

Distance units are calculated as follows:

at least 3 but less than 4 miles	:	1 unit
at least 4 but less than 5 miles	:	4 units
at least 5 but less than 6 miles	:	6 units
at least 6 but less than 7 miles	:	8 units
at least 7 but less than 8 miles	:	10 units
each additional mile or part of a mile	:	2 additional units.

Walking units will be added to these for that part of the route which has to be walked. The distance is measured from the point where a GP leaves a normal two-wheel-drive car to walk to the patient's home under normal winter conditions.

Walking units are calculated as follows:

at least a quarter but less than half a mile	:	3 units
at least half but less than three-quarters of a mile	:	6 units
at least three-quarters but less than one mile	:	9 units
each additional quarter or part of a quarter of a mile	:	3 additional units.

Blocked route units will be credited if the normal route from the GP's main surgery is regularly liable to be blocked owing to flooding or other severe weather conditions. Three units will be credited for each patient affected whatever the distance from the main surgery.

The Central Advisory Committee on Rural Practice Payments advises the Secretary of State for Health on which areas should be designated as special districts, because climatic and geographical conditions are such that not only are there difficulties of access for which walking units are given but there are also exceptional difficulties in travelling by road. Doctors will be notified by the FHSA of special districts and will receive four units per patient in the district regardless of distance from the surgery.

The FHSA maintains a register of schools, hospitals and other institutions where there are normally more than 25 patients registered. The units to be credited for these patients will be at half the prescribed rate. A list of those institutions is notifed to the GPs concerned. Patients in smaller institutions attract units at the full rate.

Units to be credited for patients not on a GP's list

Credit for units relating to temporary residents, emergency visits and patients receiving immediately necessary treatment will be given. Details are set out in paragraphs 43.14 and 43.15 of the Red Book.

Rural practice payments not based on units

Any GP can claim refunds of out-of-pocket expenses actually and necessarily incurred in travelling to visit a patient if the FHSA is satisfied that the expenses were of an exceptional nature (e.g. ferry charges, boat hire charges or toll charges). Where it is not possible for a GP to produce receipts, a certified statement of expenditure will be required.

12 Maternity medical services

THE fees paid for maternity medical services (MMS) are listed in the Red Book. A doctor *not* included in the obstetric list providing these services to his or her own patients is paid a lower level of fees than one who is included. In addition, the obstetrically approved doctor can accept women for MMS who are not on his or her ordinary list of patients. To gain admission to the obstetric list, a GP must have his or her obstetric experience approved by the local FHSA, or on appeal by the Secretary of State for Health.

How does a GP gain admission to the obstetric list?

The criteria determining entry to the obstetric list are in Schedule 5, Part I, of the NHS (General Medical Services) Regulations.

The most common qualification is to have held a six months' resident appointment in a hospital maternity unit in the European Community.

Less commonly, approval is given for experience in a maternity unit under consultant supervision during six consecutive months in the two years prior to the application. This particular entry criterion specifies how many normal deliveries, abnormal confinements and clinics a GP should have attended.

If a GP has undertaken a six months' obstetric post more than 10 years prior to applying, he or she should within the previous five years have attended a week's refresher course, or spent not less than two weeks as a resident obstetric officer in a maternity unit under consultant supervision.

There are four other entry criteria. If, when applying for inclusion in the obstetric list, a GP is already included in another FHSA's obstetric list, the application will be accepted. Similarly, if during the previous two years a doctor has been included in an obstetric list because of having held a resident six month post, the application will also be accepted. If a GP can demonstrate having been in obstetric practice in the UK and attending not less than 100 maternity cases over the previous five years, during the care of which cases he or she was responsible for ante-natal care in all and the supervision of labour and puerperium in at least 50, he or she will be accepted. Finally, the FHSA has the power to approve an application, after consultation with the LMC, if the GP's experience does not meet any of these criteria but is considered acceptable.

> **Box 12.1: Qualifying for the obstetric list**
>
> - six months' post
> - attendance at a consultant unit during six consecutive months
> - on another FHSA obstetric list
> - on an obstetric list during previous two years
> - previous obstetric experience
> - FHSA approval of previous experience

Ante-natal care fees

There are three levels of fee, and payments are not affected if the patient receives hospital care. They are paid if she is confined after the 24th week, or earlier if a live birth results. The different fees are:

- for a woman booking up to the 16th week of pregnancy
- for a woman booking from the 17th to the 30th week of pregnancy
- for a woman booking from the 31st week of pregnancy.

The date of booking is taken as the date on which the woman signs the acceptance application in Part II of form FP24/24A.

Miscarriage fee

If a woman's pregnancy ends during or before the 24th week and does not result in a live birth, a miscarriage fee is paid for any MMS provided.

Abortion

Arranging a therapeutic abortion is part of general medical services. However, if the need for an abortion arises after the patient has been accepted for MMS, a miscarriage fee is paid for any maternity services given prior to the decision that there should be an abortion. Post-operative care of a woman after an abortion does *not* qualify for post-natal care fees.

Confinement fee

This fee is paid for providing MMS during confinement and covers cases where a GP is called during labour to a patient not booked for MMS with the GP.

Premature confinement

A premature confinement after the 24th week, or at any other time if it results in a live birth, is treated as a confinement at full term and the appropriate fees are paid.

Post-natal care fees

The complete fee

A GP who provides MMS to a mother and child throughout the 14 day period immediately after confinement and carries out a full post-natal examination at or about six weeks after confinement, is paid the complete post-natal care fee. The full post-natal examination must normally be undertaken within 12 weeks of confinement. The complete fee will still be paid if the patient is confined in a hospital other than a GP unit, provided the woman leaves hospital – either to return home or to a GP maternity unit – not later than the second day after delivery.

The partial fee

A fee is paid to a GP for each attendance to give medical care to either the mother or her child during the 14 days after the birth, **but** fees are only paid for a maximum of five such attendances. A fee is also paid for a full post-natal examination at or about six weeks after confinement. This is paid if the examination is carried out up to 12 weeks after confinement. However, if a GP submits a claim for a fee, for an examination carried out later than 12 weeks, before paying the fee, the FHSA needs to be satisfied that the doctor has carried it out as soon as possible and has made reasonable efforts to undertake the examination between six and 12 weeks after confinement. The Department of Health has advised FHSAs that no payment should be made for an examination carried out within four weeks of confinement, and that a case would have to be made for payment sooner than six weeks after the confinement. It is important to emphasize that where a patient has been confined either at home or in hospital and requires medical attendance *beyond* the fourteenth day after her confinement, her own GP should provide this as part of general medical services.

What can be claimed if a post-natal examination is not undertaken?

If a GP has otherwise provided complete care, but because of circumstances beyond the doctor's control the post-natal examination has not been carried out, the FHSA may pay the full fee if satisfied that the doctor made 'reasonable efforts' to undertake the examination. Efforts accepted by a FHSA as reasonable might include two letters from the GP to the patient requesting her to attend the surgery for the examination, followed by either a request to the patient through a health visitor or midwife, or a call by the doctor at the patient's home.

Complete MMS fee

The complete MMS fee is paid to a GP who provides complete MMS during pregnancy, confinement and the post-natal period and carries out a full post-natal examination at or about six weeks after confinement. This examination should normally be carried out no later than 12 weeks after confinement. If a GP provides complete MMS to a woman and has accepted her at least six weeks before confinement, the full fee is paid.

Fee for second practitioner giving an anaesthetic

If a GP providing MMS calls a second doctor to give an anaesthetic, an additional fee is paid. The first doctor will still be entitled to that fee if for good professional reasons the second practitioner carries out the delivery and the GP who called him or her administers the anaesthetic. An anaesthetic fee is *not* payable if the anaesthetic is administered by a trainee GP for his or her trainer or the trainer's partner or assistant. Normally, only one fee is paid for a particular confinement, even if an anaesthetic is administered more than once. If, exceptionally, two separate and distinct attendances are necessary to administer an anaesthetic, a further fee is paid.

Box 12.2: MMS: specific fees payable
- complete services
- ante-natal care
- miscarriage
- confinement
- post-natal care
- for second practitioner giving an anaesthetic

Second opinion

A GP referring a patient to a consultant for a second opinion is entitled to the appropriate fees so long as he or she retains responsibility for the patient's maternity care.

What happens if a patient accepted for maternity care receives MMS from another doctor?

There may be circumstances in which a patient accepted by a GP for maternity care receives care from another GP; for instance if she lives temporarily in another area. When this occurs, the total amount paid is limited to either the fee for complete MMS or a smaller fee reflecting the actual services provided. For example, if a woman resides in another area for some time and a doctor in that area provides some MMS care then the main or 'responsible' FHSA may agree with the 'temporary' FHSA that the fees are divided proportionately between the two GPs according to the care provided (*see* Box 12.3). A similar approach is adopted if a woman moves permanently during maternity care, whether within an FHSA area or to another area.

How to claim

Claims should be made to the FHSA covering the area in which the patient lives. GPs on the obstetric list should use form FP24, and those not on the obstetric list form FP24A. Part II of the form (application for services) must be completed and signed by the patient and Part III by the doctor. (Part II contains a special certificate for the doctor to use if he or she attends a woman in an emergency and it is undesirable to ask for her signature.)

Normally, the GP's certificate on the claim form is sufficient evidence of services having been provided, but in cases of doubt the FHSA may make enquiries before authorizing payment. Thus, if the FHSA (after consulting the LMC) is not satisfied that complete MMS were provided, it may pay instead the appropriate partial care fees.

Completing the claim forms

Forms FP24 and FP24A should be completed accurately and submitted promptly. Form FP24 is shown in Fig. 12.1, and attention is drawn to those parts of the form which often lead to queries.

Box 12.3: Example of apportionment of fees between two GPs providing MMS to one woman

Both GPs on the Obstetric List

Expected date of confinement 16 October 1992

Dr A: Patient booked for MMS 25 April 1992 (15th week)
      Patient subsequently moved temporarily
Dr B: Patient booked for MMS 5 July 1992 (25th week)
      Patient returned home 38th week
Dr A: Care during confinement on 15 October 1992
      + post-natal care
      + post-natal examination at 6th week after confinement

Payment for ante-natal care

			Dr A	Dr B
1st level	Dr A:	(15th week)	£21.50	
2nd level	Dr A:	8/13 × £21.45	£13.20	
	Dr B:	5/13 × £21.45 (25th week)		£ 8.25
3rd level	Dr A:	2/9 × £42.95	£ 9.54	
	Dr B:	7/9 × £42.95		£33.41
			£44.24	£41.66

Total payment made: £85.90

Payment for confinement and post-natal care

Dr A:

Care during confinement				£36.55
Complete post-natal:	(i)	5 visits @ £4.90 during 14 days puerperium		£24.50
	(ii)	post-natal pelvic examination at or about the 6th week		£12.05
				£73.10

Dr A is paid   £117.34
Dr B is paid   £ 41.66

Total fees paid   £159.00

NB: For apportionment of ante-natal fees:
1st level (£85.90–£64.40) £21.50
2nd level (£64.40–£42.95) £21.45
3rd level   £42.95

                     £85.90

NATIONAL HEALTH SERVICE   MATERNITY MEDICAL SERVICES

PART I

(to be detached and given to the patient)

To ....

I accept your application to receive maternity medical services from me.

Your expected date of confinement is ....

Date ....   Doctor's signature..

PART II

PATIENT'S APPLICATION FOR SERVICES

(Tick appropriate box)

Dr...

A   I wish to receive maternity medical services from you. I have not made arrangements for these services with another doctor.   ☐

B   I wish to receive maternity medical services from you. I have cancelled arrangements

made with Dr..

of ....   ☐

C   I wish to receive maternity medical services from you whilst temporarily residing at:

....

....   ☐

I have made arrangements for maternity medical services in my home area with

Dr...

....

D   I have received maternity medical services from you in an emergency.   ☐

Patient's full name ....
(in block letters)

Home address ....

....

Former name..   N.H.S. No. ❶
                                                          or Date of Birth

Date................................   Patient's signature..

DOCTOR'S CERTIFICATE

(EMERGENCY ATTENDANCE FOR MISCARRIAGE)

I certify that in the circumstances I thought it desirable, in the patient's interest, not to ask her for a signature.

Date................................   Doctor's signature..

Form FP24

Figure 12.1 Form FP24.   *continued*

MATERNITY BENEFITS

There are cash benefits for mothers under the National Insurance Scheme which must be claimed within certain time limits. You are strongly advised to get Leaflet N.I. 17A and the necessary claim form from your local Maternity and Child Health Clinic, or from your local Department of Health and Social Security office not later than 14 weeks before your baby is expected.

PRESCRIPTION CHARGES AND WELFARE MILK AND VITAMINS

An expectant mother can apply on Part 1 of the Certificate of Pregnancy (Form FW8) for a prescription charge exemption certificate covering the period of her pregnancy and until her child is one year old. Details are given on Part 2 of Form FW8 and in leaflet MV11 (obtainable from Post Offices, local Department of Health and Social Security offices and local Maternity and Child Health Clinics) of how to claim free milk and vitamins.

PART III
DOCTOR'S CERTIFICATE AND CLAIM FOR PAYMENT
(*References are to paragraphs in the Statement of Fees and Allowances*)

(*Tick appropriate box*)

I certify that..(*patient's name*)

(expected date of confinement ......**②**......) had a miscarriage on ......**❸**...... ☐
was confined on .... ☐

at home .... ☐

In the GP Unit at ......**❹**...................................... Hospital ☐
In.. Hospital ☐

I further certify that I provided the services indicated below and that I had regard to and was guided by authoritative medical opinion as set out in paragraphs 31.2 and paragraph 31/Schedule 3.

(i) Complete Maternity Medical Services **❺**.................. Paras 31.7 to 31.8 ☐

(ii) Ante-natal care

Note: the date of booking is the date on which Parts I and II are completed

(a) Patient booked up to 16th week of pregnancy .... Para 31.9 ☐

(b) Patient booked from 17th week to 30th week

of pregnancy .... Para 31.9 ☐

(c) Patient booked from 31st week of pregnancy .... Para 31.9 ☐

(iii) Miscarriage .... Para 31.10 ☐

(iv) Care during the confinement........**❻**.......... Para 31.11 ☐

(v) Complete Post-Natal Care (Date of Hospital Discharge ...**❼**...) Para 31.12 ☐

(vi) Partial Post-Natal Care .... Para 31.13 ☐

(a) date of each attendance

(b) date of full post-natal examination ....**❽**....
(vii) Other services as described in the attached note................... ☐

(viii) Date of last service to patient...
(to be completed where only ante-natal care or only complete post-natal care is given.)

I claim payment for the above services.. ☐

I also claim payment for the employment as anaesthetist of Dr............................ ☐
Paras 31.15 to 31.16

Date.................... Doctor's signature..

Fees approved for payment £

Figure 12.1. Form FP24. Key:

[1] please enter correct NHS number;
[2] please enter this date other than when claiming for post-natal care only;
[3] it is important that these dates are *clearly* entered as appropriate;
[4] please enter these sections correctly because different fees are payable;
[5] this section must be completed when complete care is provided;
[6] this section should be completed *only* when a woman has been confined at home or in a GP unit;
[7] this section should be completed *only* when a woman is confined in hospital (other than a GP unit) for less than 48 hours;
[8] this section should be completed when partial care is given.

The GP's responsibilities

The Regulations specify the arrangements and conditions under which MMS are provided.

Services to a woman living permanently in a GP's practice area

A GP who has agreed to provide MMS for a woman is responsible for ensuring that she receives all necessary medical services during pregnancy, confinement and the post-natal period. This obligation applies from when she is accepted for maternity care until 14 days after confinement. However, where a woman is booked into a hospital for confinement, the hospital staff are responsible for her care during that period (unless she is in a GP maternity unit to which the GP has access). The GP is also responsible for making a full post-natal examination at or about six weeks after confinement and normally no later than 12 weeks after, other than in exceptional circumstances as explained on pages 58 and 59.

If a pregnancy ends in a miscarriage, the GP is responsible for providing care from when the woman is accepted for MMS until the miscarriage.

If a patient moves out of a GP's practice area, unless the GP agrees to continue care, he or she is responsible for her care only from when she is accepted for maternity care until she leaves the area.

Services for a woman living temporarily in a GP's practice area

If a GP accepts a woman for maternity care who is living temporarily in the practice area, the doctor's responsibility for her care is the same as if she lived there permanently. The doctor is also responsible for advising a woman on how to arrange continuing treatment if she leaves the area.

Good maternal and early neonatal care

A practitioner providing maternity care is required to certify that in providing services he or she has taken account of modern authoritative medical opinion.

13 Contraceptive services

Two types of fee are paid for contraceptive services: an ordinary fee and an intrauterine device fee. These are paid at annual rates representing payment for services over a 12 month period. FHSAs pay quarterly ordinary fees of one-quarter of the annual amount. Intrauterine device fees are also paid quarterly, but the first payment is at a higher rate than the other three quarterly payments to reflect the additional work involved in fitting a device. Any woman, irrespective of whether she is registered for general medical services, can apply to receive contraceptive services.

Payment arrangements

The ordinary fee

This is paid when GPs accept a patient, give advice and conduct any necessary examination, where appropriate prescribe drugs or an occlusive cap, and provide any necessary follow-up care. GPs can also claim the fee if they help the patient to choose a method of contraception and accept responsibility for any necessary aftercare, even though the advice may be to attend an NHS clinic for the fitting of an occlusive cap or intrauterine device. This means that even if a woman attends the surgery and advice is given about a male contraceptive or vasectomy, GPs may still claim if they accept responsibility for the aftercare of the female patient.

Box 13.1: Payment of the ordinary fee

This is paid when GPs:

- accept a patient, give contraceptive advice, conduct any examination, where appropriate prescribe drugs or an occlusive cap, and provide follow-up treatment
- help to determine choice of contraception and accept responsibility for aftercare

---

Intrauterine device

GPs can claim the intrauterine device fee for services provided to a woman during the 12 month period starting on the day she applies to have the device fitted. The fee is paid only if the GP, or a partner or an assistant, fits the device and gives all necessary aftercare including any replacement for the next 12 months. It is not possible to claim this fee in addition to the ordinary fee. Twelve months after fitting, the ordinary fee will become payable for any period during which a device is not fitted or replaced. If the device is replaced, the intrauterine device fee becomes payable again for a further 12 months. If the device is replaced within 12 months, this is deemed to be part of the aftercare and no further intrauterine device fee is paid.

Box 13.2: Payment of intrauterine device fee

This is paid when a GP fits an intrauterine device and provides aftercare for a period of 12 months

---

Temporary resident patients

A patient who is a temporary resident can also be provided with contraceptive services and the GP who accepts the patient will be paid one-quarter of the annual fee. However, if an intrauterine device is fitted or replaced, the GP receives one-half of the annual intrauterine device fee.

How to claim

Claims should be on form FP1001 for the ordinary contraceptive fee and form FP1002 if an intrauterine device has been fitted. Both forms must be signed by both the patient and GP. A claim for a temporary resident patient should be made on form FP1003, and if an intrauterine device has been fitted or replaced the doctor should state this in Part II of the form.

At the end of 12 months, a new claim must be sent to the FHSA for each patient for whom contraceptive services continue to be provided. If a patient comes to the surgery for contraceptive services within one month of the date on which the 12 month period will end, a new form can be completed and submitted to the FHSA which will accept it as taking effect from the end of the 12 month period. If a patient does not attend at about the time the 12 month period ends but does so within 18 months of the first claim, a GP can still claim that service has been continuous and the FHSA will pay retrospectively for the missing quarters. For instance, if a patient was first accepted in May 1992 but does not attend the surgery again until September 1993 seeking renewal of contraceptive services, the claim can be regarded as being submitted in May 1993. A different doctor can sign the second claim if he or she is the successor to the GP making the first claim or the doctors are partners.

If a GP accepts a woman for ordinary services but later decides to fit an intrauterine device, a new claim should be made on form FP1002 which will supersede the form FP1001, and a further claim will become due 12 months after the insertion of the intrauterine device.

A GP will cease to be paid for a patient as soon as an FHSA receives a subsequent claim from another doctor. Claim forms should be sent on a regular basis to the FHSA.

The FHSA calculates the current claims on the first day of each quarter and advises each doctor of the number of patients involved. The GP has 10 days to challenge the figure; if no challenge is made within that time, there will be no further opportunity to do so.

14 Child health surveillance

A doctor who wishes to be paid for child health surveillance should apply to the FHSA to be included on its child health surveillance list.

A GP on the child health surveillance list is paid a fee for each child under five years of age for whom services are provided in accordance with the programme agreed between the FHSA and the District Health Authority (DHA) for the area where the doctor practises.

Child health surveillance patient list

A GP on the child health surveillance list should inform the FHSA on form FP/CHS of each child for whom he or she has undertaken to provide surveillance. The FHSA maintains a separate list of these children, in addition to the normal general medical services patient list. This list may include children on the doctor's normal list together with those on the lists of partners or other doctors with whom he or she works in a group practice.

Level and method of payment

There is one level of fee and this is paid on the first day of each quarter according to the information provided by the doctor on form FP/CHS. Payment is made whether or not any particular service has been provided for that child during the preceding quarter. Payment ceases when the child reaches the age of five years.

15 Minor surgery

To claim a fee for this work a GP must be included in the FHSA's minor surgery list. It is paid for minor surgery sessions provided for his or her own patients or those of partners or group members.

No more than three payments can be made to a GP in the same quarter, except that if the GP is in a partnership or group practice, more payments may be claimed provided that the total number paid in any quarter does not exceed three times the number of partners or members of the group on the medical list on the first day of that quarter.

What is a session?

A session consists of five surgical procedures; they may be performed either in a single clinic or on separate occasions during the same quarter. Procedures will count towards a session if they meet the following criteria:

- they are included in this list:

Injections	intra-articular
	peri-articular
	varicose veins
	haemorrhoids
Aspirations	joints
	cysts
	bursae
	hydrocele
Incisions	abscesses
	cysts
	thrombosed piles
Excisions	sebaceous cysts
	lipoma
	skin lesions for histology
	intradermal naevi, papillomata, dermatofibromata and similar conditions
	warts
	removal of toe nails (partial and complete)
Curette cautery and cryocautery	warts and verrucae
	other skin lesions e.g. molluscum contagiosum

Other   removal of foreign bodies
                         nasal cautery

- they are performed by a doctor on the FHSA's minor surgery list
- any other person assisting in a procedure is suitably trained or experienced
  for the task.

Minor surgery list

A doctor who wants to do minor surgery should apply to the FHSA for inclusion on the minor surgery list. The qualifying criteria are specified in the Regulations.

How to claim payment

Claims should be made on form FP/MS which records basic information about the patient's doctor, the doctor carrying out the procedure and the date and type of procedure. FHSAs check the validity of claims.

16 Restricted services and limited lists

A doctor admitted to the medical list to provide only maternity medical services

A doctor included on an FHSA's list to provide only MMS is entitled to claim fees for those services. It may also be possible to claim direct reimbursement for surgery premises and practice staff. A doctor who incurs expenses on premises or staff will receive direct reimbursement if payment can be justified by the amount of NHS work undertaken. (An application form REST2 should be sent to the FHSA together with the relevant PREM and PS forms relating to the premises and staff for which reimbursement is being claimed.) If the amount of work does not justify payment at the full rate, a lower rate may be paid. A doctor who is building up a practice providing only MMS can expect to be given special consideration.

The scheme for additional payments during sickness also applies to a doctor providing only MMS. The definition of the word 'service' in the relevant Red Book paragraph includes MMS only. A woman doctor claiming payments during confinement should apply via the FHSA to the Secretary of State for Health.

A doctor can also be paid for providing a dispensing service to patients in accordance with the rural dispensing arrangements.

A doctor admitted to the medical list for the provision of contraceptive services only

A doctor may be admitted to the medical list to provide contraceptive services only and will be paid for doing so.

Similar arrangements to those described in the section above on the provision of MMS only, apply to rent and rates and practice staff reimbursements and additional payments during sickness and confinement.

Payments may be made for the supply of contraceptive drugs and appliances.

A limited list practitioner

A doctor whose list is limited to the staff of one or more hospitals or a similar institution in which he or she is employed, or to patients registered in, or connected with, one or more schools or other institutions, is not entitled to a Basic Practice Allowance (BPA) or any of the other allowances additional to the BPA. He or she will not be able to claim a postgraduate education allowance or certain direct payments for expenses.

However, a limited list doctor is entitled to standard capitation fees (including the higher fees for elderly patients) which will be abated by 10%, and if he or she is included in the child health surveillance list, the appropriate fees for this work will be paid.

The limited list GP is also able to claim fees for special services, although a night visit fee will not be paid for any visit to a resident in an institution where the doctor resides.

A GP with a limited list may claim rent and rates and practice staff reimbursements. The level of these payments will depend on the amount of NHS work undertaken. Special consideration will be given to a doctor with a limited list in partnership with other doctors providing unrestricted services, whose rent and rates and practice staff reimbursements have been abated because of that doctor's private income.

Additional payments during sickness may also be paid; a doctor with a limited list of at least 1200 patients will qualify in full for additional payments during sickness. If he or she has less than 1200 patients, the payment will be scaled down to a minimum of a 20% payment for 400 patients. No payment will be made if there are less than 400 patients on the list.

Claims for additional payments during confinement will be considered by the Secretary of State in consultation with the General Medical Services Committee of the British Medical Association.

GPs relieved before 1 April 1990 of the liability to provide certain services

A doctor who was permitted by an FPC's allocation committee to be relieved of the responsibility to have patients assigned to him or her under the allocation scheme will continue to receive standard capitation fees, deprivation payments and child health surveillance fees in full but the basic practice allowance will be cut by 25%.

A doctor who has contracted to provide services for his or her patients out of hours and has obtained the consent of the allocation committee to be exempted from liability to answer emergency calls during those hours from patients who:

- are not on his or her list; or
- are not temporary residents for whom he or she is responsible; or
- have not been accepted by him or her for the provision of maternity medical services,

will have the basic practice allowance reduced by 5%.

A doctor admitted to the medical list solely to treat patients as temporary residents

A doctor may be included on an FHSA medical list for the sole purpose of treating temporary residents at the rates and on the conditions authorized by the Secretary of State. No other payments or reimbursements will be made.

A doctor admitted to the medical list for the provision of child health surveillance services only

A doctor may be admitted to the medical list to provide only child health surveillance services and will receive CHS fees only.

Arrangements for reimbursing the costs of premises and staff are similar to those applying to doctors providing MMS or contraceptive services only. Additional payments during sickness and confinement may also be claimed.

A doctor admitted to the medical list for the provision of minor surgery services only

A GP can apply for admission to an FHSA's minor surgery list and be paid for undertaking minor surgery work. He or she can claim help towards the cost of premises and staff, but cannot receive payments during sickness or confinement. Claims can also be made for the provision of drugs and appliances.

⌐17 The registration fee

A doctor who carries out the examination procedures specified in the terms of service within three months of inviting a patient for examination who has been newly accepted onto the doctor's personal list will be eligible for a registration fee.

If the examination procedure is carried out more than three months after the date of the patient's acceptance, the FHSA will still pay a fee if it is satisfied that the doctor carried out the procedure as soon as possible, and had made all reasonable efforts to do so within three months of the patient's acceptance but was prevented by factors beyond his or her control.

When a doctor succeeds to a practice vacancy, or otherwise becomes responsible for a significant number of new patients within a short period, he or she may apply to the FHSA for permission to defer the obligation to invite patients for a registration check for up to two years.

No fee is paid for:

- a child under five years of age at the time of joining the list
- a patient who immediately before joining the list was a patient of a partner, and who participated in a 'registration' consultation during the 12 months prior to the date of acceptance
- an examination carried out more than 12 months after the date of invitation for examination.

Method of payment

Claims should be submitted to the FHSA on form FP/RF. The FHSA may check with patients that registration checks have been carried out.

18 Health promotion and chronic disease management

For many years, GPs have been involved in opportunistic health promotion, planned call and recall of patients for preventive care and the planned management of patients with chronic diseases. Until 1990, this work was undertaken as part of general medical services, without any specific payment or any additional funding; the profession was rewarded within average net remuneration.

However, the new contract introduced on 1 April 1990 made health promotion a specific obligation under GPs' terms of service. GPs were obliged to give 'advice, where appropriate, to a patient in connection with the patient's general health, and in particular about the significance of diet, exercise, the use of tobacco, the consumption of alcohol and the misuse of drugs or solvents', as well as to offer 'consultations and, where appropriate, physical examinations for the purpose of . . . reducing the risk of disease or injury'.

In addition, GPs were able to claim fees for health promotion clinics. Well-person clinics, anti-smoking clinics, clinics for alcohol control, dietary advice, exercise counselling, stress management, heart disease prevention, and the care of patients with diabetes or asthma generally qualified for payment, and other clinics could also be submitted for approval by FHSAs. So long as the purpose of and arrangements for clinics were approved by the FHSA, there was no limit on the number of clinics for which GPs could claim.

A rapid growth in expenditure on clinics resulted: in 1990–91, £50 million was paid to GPs in Great Britain by way of health promotion clinic fees, in the second year of the scheme £73 million was paid out, and in the third year £80 million was claimed. Although collectively GPs were doing more and more work for the same total pool of money, individual GPs sought to maximize their own income by undertaking increasing numbers of clinics, and the level of activity only stopped climbing with the imposition of a moratorium on 1 July 1992. If a moratorium had not been imposed, there was every reason to suppose that the amount GPs were earning from health promotion clinics would have gone on increasing, with the result that GPs would have been paid less and less for the rest of their work. Indeed, the growth in health promotion clinics was a major factor in the destabilization of the GP remuneration system which occurred after the introduction of the 1990 contract.

This clinic activity was very unevenly distributed among practices, with no activity being recorded in many and substantial amounts in others. The distribution could not easily be explained by the needs of patients, and the problem was undoubtedly compounded by the application of differing approval criteria by different FHSAs and Health Boards. The profession collectively said that it felt cheapened and demoralized by, and cynical about, the operation of the clinic system, coupled with GPs' obligation under the Regulations introduced in 1990 to offer a consultation to patients between the ages of 16 and 75 years who had not been seen in general practice within the preceding three years. There was thus considerable pressure for change in the contractual arrangements governing health promotion, and protracted negotiations were undertaken in order to achieve a new system, and to supersede the requirement for GPs to invite non-attenders for three-yearly checks.

The intention was to fashion a system with greater accountability, greater equitability and greater scientific validity, as well as greater professional freedom, recognizing in particular the value of opportunistic intervention. Both Government and profession wanted to see resources targeted on proven activities which would be of greatest benefit to patients. The negotiations took place within the framework set by the White Paper *The Health of the Nation*, published in July 1992, and the equivalent Scottish and Welsh strategic guidance, and it was decided to focus health promotion activity on the prevention of coronary heart disease and stroke.

It was also seen that health promotion activities had to be appropriate to local needs and circumstances, and to reflect dialogue between FHSAs, LMCs and GPs. FHSAs and DHAs would need to make information available to practices on other relevant local health promotion activities, so that unnecessary duplication could be avoided.

The payment arrangements would need to encourage the wider availability to patients of consistent health promotion programmes, to produce a more equitable distribution of income to GPs, and to deliver a more predictable year-on-year allocation of resources to health promotion activities. It was therefore decided during the negotiating process that health promotion and chronic disease management should be paid for from a pool within a pool: within the total amount of money available for GPs' remuneration, a fixed sum should be set aside for these activities. The size of that pool was to be similar to the amount spent on clinics during the third year of their operation. Such an approach had the virtues of stopping further devaluation of the amount GPs were paid for the rest of their work (including the treatment of sick patients), of circumscribing the level of total health promotion activity, and of making it easier to resist the inclusion of additional activities in the work of GPs without the provision of new money to pay for them. Additionally, the risk of overpayments being made to the profession – which would then need to be clawed back under the Review Body's balancing arrangements – would be controlled by a system of annual bidding and fee adjustment.

The new system which resulted from this negotiating context was introduced on 1 July 1993.

The prevention of coronary heart disease and stroke

The main focus for the health promotion element of the new arrangements is coronary heart disease and stroke. The scheme is structured in three bands, so as to encourage practices to deliver progressively more comprehensive lifestyle-based preventive care to their practice population.

Band one (*see* Box 18.1) concentrates on the development of an age–sex register and the provision of programmes to reduce smoking. In band two (*see* Box 18.2) practices offer programmes to minimize the mortality and morbidity in patients with established coronary heart disease or stroke, or at risk from hypertension. Band three (*see* Box 18.3) includes programmes offering the full range of primary prevention of coronary heart disease and stroke.

Any practice wishing to participate in the scheme develops a programme of health promotion designed to meet its own patients' needs. FHSAs and Health Boards approve practice programmes in the light of national guidance and discussions with LMCs.

The levels of payment quoted in the Red Book are based on a GP with an average list size. The amount actually paid is determined by the GP's actual list size.

Box 18.1: Band one health promotion programme: smoking cessation

What does a practice have to do?

- develop a practice age–sex register
- collect information opportunistically on the smoking habits of the target population (those aged 15–74)
- offer advice, interventions and follow up, as appropriate, in line with modern medical opinion, relevant local factors and practice guidelines, to reduce smoking
- identify priority groups within the target population and seek to reach priority patients not presenting at the surgery
- work with other individuals or agencies who can help with smoking cessation

What level of coverage is expected?

- by the end of the first full year, a minimum of 30% of the target population should have had their smoking status recorded (22% in period 1 July 1993–31 March 1994)
- during each of the subsequent 12 month periods, there should be an increase of at least 15% up to a maximum coverage level of 80%

Box 18.2: Band two health promotion programme: minimizing mortality and morbidity from hypertension, coronary heart disease and stroke

What does a practice have to do?

- carry out regular opportunistic checks to identify patients in the target population (those aged 15–74) with previously undiscovered raised blood pressure
- maintain a register of patients with hypertension, coronary heart disease and stroke
- manage those patients, by means of lifestyle interventions whenever appropriate, in line with modern medical opinion and practice guidelines
- work with other people and agencies to achieve these aims
- **band two also subsumes activities in band one**

What level of coverage is expected?

- by the end of the first full year, a minimum of 30% of the target population should have had their smoking status and blood pressure recorded (22% in period 1 July 1993–31 March 1994)
- during each of the subsequent 12 month periods, there should be an increase of at least 15% up to maximum coverage levels of 80% for smoking status and 90% for blood pressure

---

Box 18.3: Band three health promotion programme: reducing the incidence of coronary heart disease and stroke by primary prevention

What does a practice have to do?

- collect information on smoking, blood pressure, body mass index, alcohol use, family history
- monitor diet and physical activity among patients aged 15–74 years
- offer lifestyle advice, other interventions and follow up, taking into account modern medical opinion, local factors and practice guidelines
- focus activity on priority groups and seek to reach patients who do not attend surgery
- work with other people and agencies
- **band three also subsumes activities in bands one and two**

What level of coverage is expected?

- by the end of the first full year a minimum of 30% of the target population should have had their smoking status recorded, 30% their blood pressure recorded (22% during the period 1 July 1993–31 March 1994), 20% their body mass index, alcohol consumption and family history of CHD/stroke recorded (15% during the period 1 July 1993–31 March 1994)
- during each of the subsequent 12 month periods there should be an increase of at least 15% up to maximum coverage levels of 80% for smoking status, 90% for blood pressure and 75% for body mass index, alcohol and family history

Chronic disease management: asthma and diabetes

There is separate recognition of organized programmes of care intended to help patients with asthma and diabetes. The payment is for running and managing the programme, rather than for the care of individual patients. Separate payments can be claimed for asthma or for diabetes care or both, and the payments are of fixed sums, which do not vary in accordance with list size.

Programmes must include the following elements:

- register
- call and recall
- education of newly diagnosed patients
- continuing education
- individual management plans
- regular review
- teamwork — appropriate links with appropriately trained professionals
- referral policies
- record keeping
- audit.

These requirements are set out in greater detail in boxes 18.4 and 18.5.

Box 18.4: Chronic disease management: asthma care

Practices will be expected to have a programme for caring for asthma patients.

What does a practice have to do?

- maintain a register of all asthma patients
- ensure that systematic call and recall of patients on the register is taking place, in either hospital or GP setting
- give advice to newly diagnosed patients or their carers
- ensure all asthma patients (or their carers) receive continuing education, including supervising inhaler technique
- prepare with the patient an individual management plan
- regularly review the patients (including peak flow measurements), generally every six months, but more or less frequently as required
- ensure any health professionals involved in the care of asthma patients are appropriately trained
- refer patients to other services as required
- maintain adequate records and audit the care programme

Box 18.5: Chronic disease management: diabetes care

Practices will be expected to have a programme for caring for diabetic patients.

What does a practice have to do?

- maintain a register of all diabetic patients
- ensure that systematic call and recall of patients on the register is taking place, in either hospital or GP setting
- give advice to newly diagnosed patients or their carers
- ensure all diabetic patients (or their carers) receive continuing education
- prepare with the patient an individual management plan
- ensure that on initial diagnosis and at least annually, a full review of the patient's health is carried out, including checks for potential complications and a review of the patient's own monitoring records
- work together with other professionals (e.g. dietitians and chiropodists) where appropriate
- ensure any health professionals involved in the care of diabetic patients are appropriately trained
- refer patients to other services and supportive agencies as required, using locally agreed referral guidelines where these exist
- maintain adequate records and audit the care programme

Transitional arrangements and priorities reflecting local circumstances

Despite the concentration of the care programme on coronary heart disease, stroke, asthma and diabetes, and despite the intention to ensure that health promotion is appropriately and adequately resourced, the new scheme is also intended to allow the addressing of other locally agreed priorities, flowing either from central strategic intentions or from the identification of particular local needs. Many practices had already been undertaking worthwhile activity outside the scope of the core programme, and further developments should be encouraged when circumstances and resources permit.

In the first nine months of the new scheme's operation, from 1 July 1993 to 31 March 1994, transitional payments will be available to those practices offering a band three health promotion programme, which were earning more money under the previous health promotion clinic arrangements than they can now earn from band three activities and asthma and diabetes care programmes, so long as they are carrying out an approved transitional programme. At the time of writing, practices have applied for transitional payments on form FP/HPP/3, but the precise details of how the sum set aside will be distributed to eligible GPs are under discussion.

In the second year of the scheme, from 1 April 1994 to 31 March 1995, it is intended that money will be redeployed from the transitional fund, to fund new activity within the care programmes and to resource new and existing activity within locally agreed priorities, and by the third year of the scheme, the entire transitional fund will have been redeployed in that way.

Meanwhile, in the second year of the scheme, transitional payments will continue to be paid to practices which had been receiving them from the start of the new system, but at approximately half the rate paid in the first nine months.

Again, the details of the operation of the transitional payments after 1 April 1994 and of the locally agreed priority schemes are at the time of writing under discussion between the Department of Health and the profession's negotiators.

Organization of programmes

Practices will have to apply for approval of their programmes on an annual basis, by 31 January each year, on form FP/HPP/1, and to report progress in their annual reports by 30 June. They also have to include mid-year summaries of their progress to date on form FP/HPP/2, with their applications for reapproval.

It is open to single-handed doctors and two doctor practices to collaborate with others to organize and offer a joint programme if they wish.

The information in the Red Book about health promotion and chronic disease management has been supplemented by extensive guidance for regional authorities, FHSAs, LMCs and practices, sent out by the Department of Health on 12 January 1993 (FHSL(93)3). The guidance emphasizes that the information required by FHSAs in order to determine whether the programme meets the Red Book criteria should not be excessive or repetitive. Many practices may wish to refer in their applications to protocols or guidelines already approved under the old clinic arrangements, or to readily available national clinical guidance.

FHSAs are required to consult LMCs on the way in which the guidance from the Department of Health is followed through locally. Such consultation is required on issues arising from *The Health of the Nation* and regional, DHA and FHSA strategies for meeting Health of the Nation targets which should be taken into account in developing health promotion programmes; on local factors relevant to the development of health promotion programmes, including the selection of priority groups; on the level of coverage to be expected, and whether variations from national guidance are justified by local circumstances; and on the shared care arrangements for chronic disease management. FHSAs may also consult LMCs on the approach to be adopted in relation to borderline or unusual cases (*see* Box 18.6).

Box 18.6: Consultation with the LMC

- development of health promotion programmes in relation to *Health of the Nation* and strategic policy documents
- local factors relevant to programmes
- selection of priority groups
- level of coverage
- shared care arrangements for chronic disease management
- approach to borderline or unusual cases

The Department of Health is taking an active role centrally and through regions, in order to promote the fair and consistent application of the new arrangements throughout the country, and is encouraging dialogue at regional level between NHS management and the profession about the framework, its implementation and any inconsistencies in interpretation.

Annual reports and information requirements

The move from health promotion clinics to health promotion programmes is founded on a more population-based approach to preventive care. Some basic information on the practice population is needed to underpin these programmes, and is to be summarized in annual reports. Many practices already hold such information, but for some it will be a new task; practices without computers face a particular challenge.

The contents of annual reports have therefore been rationalized (*see* pages 27 and 29); some previous requirements have been pruned, including information about premises, staffing and referrals, so as to eliminate duplication of data available elsewhere. The aim is to concentrate on information needed to support the new programmes, building on basic information supplied by all GPs on the health of their practice population.

Additional information will be expected from GPs offering health promotion or chronic disease management programmes, including a commentary indicating whether progress on coverage levels has been as expected, whether changes in the programme have been or will be required, what audit has been carried out, and whether joint working with other individuals or agencies has occurred.

The degree of detail in which practices compile information will be influenced by whether or not they are computerized, their computer's reporting capacity, and their own needs and interests. Rates of progress towards comprehensive information gathering will vary, and in the first year of the scheme it is acceptable for practices starting from a low base to demonstrate good progress, if they cannot meet the information requirements in full.

The detailed information requirements are defined in the Red Book, while the Departmental guidance suggests methods of presenting the data. In summary, information will be collected on a head count basis – the numbers of patients given advice, offered interventions etc – rather than an activity basis – the number of clinic sessions – and will be broken down by age and sex.

Professional guidance

The Chief Medical Officer's Joint Working Group on Health Promotion, with membership from the General Medical Services Committee of the BMA, the Royal College of General Practitioners and the Department of Health commissioned from Knowledge House a resource pack on lifestyle interventions for coronary heart disease and stroke prevention, to aid GPs and other members of the primary health care team in their work of helping patients stop smoking, become more physically active, eat more healthily and drink within sensible limits. This publication, *Better Living – Better Life*, was distributed to every practice in England, Wales and Scotland in January 1993.

Additionally, the Royal College and the GMSC have developed updated professional guidelines on the management of asthma and diabetes, and the GMSC distributed to every GP in February 1993 a guide to the new health promotion package including an introduction and summary; a question and answer section; guidance on developing chronic disease management programmes; and the full text of the Department of Health's guidance on the new arrangements.

19 Night visit fees and out of hours services

Night visit fees

A GP is paid a fee for each visit both requested and made between 10 p.m. and 8 a.m. to a patient on his or her personal list, a temporary resident, or a woman for whom he or she is providing maternity medical services who is visited in connection with those services. Both the request and the visit must be made between 10 p.m. and 8 a.m. (Under the pre-1990 GP contract claims were only payable for visits both requested and made between 11 p.m. and 7 a.m.)

Claims are made on form FP81. Although the patient's signature is not required on this form, FHSAs make random checks with patients or their relatives to ensure the validity of claims. If a GP considers there are circumstances that an FHSA should be aware of before it makes a request for confirmation, these should be stated on the form.

Box 19.1: Night visit fees are paid if:

- the visit is both requested and made between 10 p.m. and 8 a.m.
- the patient is on the GP's personal list, or is a temporary resident, or has been accepted for maternity medical services

---

In certain circumstances a claim can be made for treatment given at a surgery or GP hospital, if this was in the patient's interests. A fee may also be paid for a visit to a woman in hospital to provide maternity medical services.

Level of fees

Night visit fees are at two levels. The higher fee is payable if the visit is made by any of the following:

- the practitioner with whom the patient is registered
- a partner or member of his or her group practice
- an approved assistant of the partnership or group
- an associate
- a deputy or locum who is directly employed by a practitioner or a member of the partnership or group and whose employment has been notified to the FHSA, but not where the deputy or locum made the visit on behalf of a

deputizing service with whom such a member had entered into an arrangement approved under the terms of service

- a trainee practitioner employed by a practitioner or a member of the partnership or group
- a single-handed GP or a GP in a group or partnership who is part of a local non-commercial rota which includes GPs, outside of his or her group or partnership, who may themselves be single-handed, partners or working in a group, whose number does not exceed 10 and who have agreed to provide out of hours cover for each other.

In all other cases the lower fee will be paid.

Box 19.2: Level of fees

- there are two levels of night visit fees
- a higher fee is paid for visits by the GP with whom the patient is registered, a partner, group member, assistant, associate, deputy, locum, trainee, or a member of a non-commercial rota of up to 10 practitioners

---

In defining 'ten practitioner rotas', the Red Book states that the GPs do not need to work from the same surgery and explains how they should notify the FHSA of the members of the rota. A practitioner may not be in more than one rota at a time.

If more than one patient is seen on a visit to one location, payment is made in accordance with the following formula:

- two patients seen on one visit to one location: one full fee for each patient
- additional one, two or three patients: one half for each additional patient
- for each patient seen after the first five: one tenth of the full fee.

A school, hotel, holiday camp or similar establishment is regarded as one location. If a GP considers that this formula does not provide fair compensation, the FHSA may pay at a higher rate no greater than one full fee per patient.

Practitioners relieved of the responsibility to provide out of hours services

A few GPs do not have to provide out of hours services to their patients under a preserved right specified in paragraph 18(2) of the terms of service. Those who had such relief on 31 March 1990 will continue to enjoy this whilst they remain on the FHSA list. Practitioners who take on responsibility for out of hours services to the patients of these 'opted out' doctors receive a capitation addition for each patient.

20 Temporary residents

A GP who treats a temporary resident is paid a fee:

- at a lower rate if the temporary resident expects to remain in the area for not more than 15 days from when the GP first provides treatment
- at a higher rate if the temporary resident expects to remain in the area for more than 15 days.

Payment is only made if the FHSA is satisifed that treatment has actually been provided. A patient is regarded as a temporary resident if in the area for more than 24 hours but less than three months.

Box 20.1: Temporary residents

- fee paid only if treatment is actually provided
- two rates of payment, depending on whether patient is in the area for less or more than 15 days from when treatment is first provided
- the patient is temporarily resident for more than 24 hours and less than three months

---

If the only treatment provided attracts an item-of-service fee for vaccination, immunization, contraceptive services, maternity medical services or the arrest of dental haemorrhage, this fee is paid instead of the temporary resident fee. A night visit fee can be claimed in addition to the temporary resident fee.

Fees are only paid if the patient is a temporary resident; they cannot be claimed for those patients permanently resident in the area whom a GP wishes to accept on only a temporary basis.

21 Fees for miscellaneous services

Emergency treatment

A GP can claim an emergency treatment fee for providing a service in an accident or other emergency to someone not registered with the practice who is staying in the area for no more than 24 hours. It is the total, not the remaining length of stay which determines whether an emergency or temporary resident fee is claimed. For example, if someone is staying in the practice area for only seven days and needs treatment on the sixth day, a temporary resident fee is paid rather than an emergency treatment fee, even if the patient is returning home within 24 hours of the consultation.

If the service includes a visit between 10 p.m. and 8 a.m., a higher emergency treatment fee is paid; a night visit claim on form FP81 should not be submitted.

Box 21.1: Emergency treatment fees
- a fee is paid if a GP provides a service to someone not registered with the practice whose total stay is less than 24 hours
- a higher rate is paid for a visit between 10 p.m. and 8 a.m.

Different services attract different levels of emergency treatment fee. If a GP considers that he or she has provided a service which is not covered by the list in the Red Book (paragraph 1, schedule 1), or an abnormal amount of time has been taken in providing the treatment, he or she may apply to the FHSA for a special fee.

If a GP provides a service to a patient of a neighbouring practice, the FHSA may deduct the payment (except the fee for a visit made between 10 p.m. and 8 a.m.) from the patient's own doctor's remuneration if he or she was not available to provide the service personally. Before doing so, the FHSA will give the doctor the opportunity to explain his or her non-attendance.

The FHSA will not pay an emergency treatment fee for a service for which it is possible to recover a fee under the Road Traffic Act, unless it is satisfied the GP has been unable to do so. A fee recovered under this Act is usually paid through the motor vehicle insurance company. A GP can ask the FHSA how to obtain payment from the insurance company, and whether an emergency treatment fee would be paid if the fee cannot be recovered.

If the only service provided attracts an item-of-service fee for vaccination, immunization, or the arrest of dental haemorrhage, an emergency treatment fee cannot be claimed.

How to claim

Form FP32 should be sent to the FHSA, and should include details of any claim for a rural practice payment.

The flow chart in Fig. 21.1 shows when temporary resident fees, emergency treatment fees or fees for immediately necessary treatment may be claimed.

Immediately necessary treatment

If a person requires treatment and the GP is unwilling to accept him or her as a patient or a temporary resident, the GP is obliged under the terms of service to provide all immediately necessary treatment. The fee for this service may be claimed on form FP106.

This fee is the same as that which would be paid for a temporary resident, even if the patient is assigned to the GP's list within three months of the date the service is provided. However, if the person is subsequently accepted as a permanent or temporary resident patient by the doctor or the doctor's partner within three months, the GP will be deemed to have accepted the patient with effect from the date that the immediately necessary treatment was provided.

A night visit fee may also be payable in addition to the immediately necessary treatment fee, as may item-of-service fees, maternity medical service fees and fees for the arrest of dental haemorrhage, although (with the exception of night visits) if the only service provided attracts an item-of-service fee, no immediately necessary treatment fee is payable.

Arrest of a dental haemorrhage

A GP who arrests a dental haemorrhage (or provides aftercare such as removing a plug or stitches) can claim a fee on form FP82. However, the GP who arrests the haemorrhage or his or her partner cannot also be paid for the aftercare. If a night visit fee is claimed for attending a patient with a dental haemorrhage, the fee for arresting the haemorrhage will **not** be paid in addition.

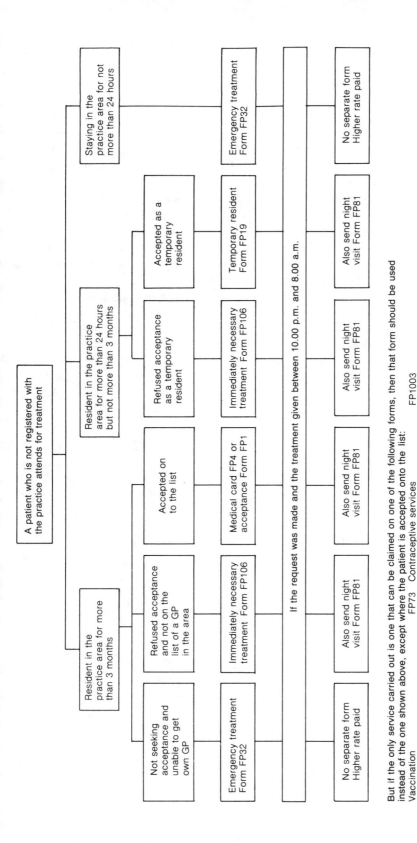

Figure 21.1 A flow chart illustrating when temporary resident fees, emergency treatment fees or fees for immediately necessary treatment may be claimed.

The content within the flow chart:

A patient who is not registered with the practice attends for treatment

Resident in the practice area for more than 3 months

- Not seeking acceptance and unable to get own GP
  - Emergency treatment Form FP32
  - No separate form Higher rate paid

- Refused acceptance and not on the list of a GP in the area
  - Immediately necessary treatment Form FP106
  - Also send night visit Form FP81

- Accepted on to the list
  - Medical card FP4 or acceptance Form FP1
  - Also send night visit Form FP81

Resident in the practice area for more than 24 hours but not more than 3 months

- Refused acceptance as a temporary resident
  - Immediately necessary treatment Form FP106
  - Also send night visit Form FP81

- Accepted as a temporary resident
  - Temporary resident Form FP19
  - Also send night visit Form FP81

Staying in the practice area for not more than 24 hours

- Emergency treatment Form FP32
  - No separate form Higher rate paid

If the request was made and the treatment given between 10.00 p.m. and 8.00 a.m.

But if the only service carried out is one that can be claimed on one of the following forms, then that form should be used instead of the one shown above, except where the patient is accepted onto the list:

Vaccination   FP73   Contraceptive services   FP1003
Arrest of dental haemorrhage   FP82
Maternity Medical Services   FP24

Service of an anaesthetist

A fee is paid to a GP if a second doctor's services are required in order to administer a general anaesthetic for any reason other than in connection with maternity medical services, when a fee is payable in accordance with the maternity services section of the Red Book.

The fee is paid whether the anaesthetic is administered by the GP responsible for the patient or by the second doctor, although a fee cannot be claimed if it is administered by a trainee or by a doctor who is doing so to enable the operation to be performed by his or her trainee. A fee is also not paid if the operation at which the anaesthetic is given is performed under arrangements made for hospital or specialist services.

If a practice makes more than 65 claims in a quarter, the FHSA will submit details to the Secretary of State, who will determine an appropriate rate of payment after consultation with the General Medical Services Committee.

Claims should be submitted on form FP31.

Cervical cytology

GPs are no longer paid item-of-service fees for cervical cytology tests; instead payment is based on a system of target payments reflecting levels of uptake.

Eligibility

A GP will receive a target payment at the higher rate if, on the first day of each quarter, at least 80% of the eligible women on his or her list, aged between 25 and 64 (21 and 60 in Scotland), have had an adequate smear (taken by any source) during a period of 5.5 years preceding the claim. Women aged 25 to 64 are defined as those born between the second day of the same quarter 65 years earlier and the first day of the quarter 40 years later. For example, on 1 October 1993, the target population of women includes those born between 2 October 1928 and 1 October 1968.

A GP will be paid a target payment at the lower rate if at least 50% of the eligible women on the partnership list have had an adequate test.

When the scheme was initially proposed, target payments were to be calculated on an individual basis for each doctor, relating solely to the women registered on his or her list. However, the scheme was subsequently modified so that target payments were calculated on a partnership basis.

The actual payment depends on the number of eligible patients, compared with those on the list of the average GP, and the number of adequate smears taken as part of general medical services as opposed to those done in DHA or private clinics.

Who is excluded from the target calculation?

Women who have had hysterectomies involving the complete removal of the cervix are excluded from the total number of women on the list when calculating coverage. GPs should notify their FHSA of the number of women in the age group who have had hysterectomies, and the number of those women who have had an adequate smear in the preceding 5.5 years, and should inform it of any new cases. No other categories of women are excluded from the calculation.

Maximum sum payable

The maximum sum payable to a GP depends on the number of eligible women aged between 25 and 64 on the partnership list, compared with the average number of such women. The average number is calculated by multiplying 430 (the number of eligible women on the average GP's list) by the number of partners. The maximum sum payable is therefore:

$$\frac{\text{number of eligible women on partnership list}}{430 \times \text{number of partners}} \quad \times \quad \begin{array}{c}\text{maximum sum payable} \\ \text{to the average GP}\end{array}$$

Calculating the payment

The GP is eligible for the whole of the relevant maximum payment if at least 80%, or 50%, of the eligible women have had adequate smear tests carried out by GPs as part of general medical services.

The smear test may have been undertaken by other doctors in the partnership or other GPs, for example if the woman was registered with another practice before joining the current GP's list. As long as the tests were adequate and carried out as part of general medical services, they are included. However, tests taken by a GP as part of work for which payment by a health authority or another source is received are excluded.

If any smears are repeated during the 5.5 year period, an adequate smear taken by a GP will take precedence over one taken by any other source for the purpose of calculating payments.

If the target is reached but the number of adequate smear tests carried out by GPs as part of general medical services is below the target number, the maximum payment is scaled down. The GP is paid that proportion of the maximum which the number of adequate tests holds to the target number.

Examples

The following two examples illustrate the target calculation and payment system.

Example 1: four-partner practice

Target calculation

Total number of eligible women aged 25–64
(hysterectomies excluded)   = 1440

Total number of women who have had an adequate smear
in the preceding 5.5 years   = 1200

$$\frac{1200}{1440} = 83.3\%$$

Higher target payment is achieved. The number of smears required to reach the higher target (the target number) is 1152 (80% of 1440).

Calculation of maximum sum payable

$$\text{Maximum sum payable} = \frac{1440 \text{ (number of eligible women on partnership list)}}{430 \text{ (number of eligible women on average list)} \times 4 \text{ (number of partners)}} \times \text{Maximum sum payable for the average practitioner (80\% level)}$$

Calculation of payment

Total number of adequate smears = 1200
of which 800 done by GP or partner
         160 done by another GP
         200 done by DHA
          40 done privately

Therefore 960 were undertaken under general medical services.

$$\text{Maximum sum payable} \times \frac{960}{1152} = \text{actual payment to each partner}$$

Example 2: three-partner practice

Target calculation

Total number of eligible women aged 25–64
(hysterectomies excluded)   = 600

Total number of women who have had an adequate smear
in the preceding 5.5 years   = 330

$$\frac{330}{600} = 55\%$$

Lower target payment is achieved. The number of smears required to reach the lower target (the target number) is 300 (50% of 600).

Calculation of maximum sum payable

$$\text{Maximum sum payable} = \frac{600}{430 \times 3} \times \text{maximum sum payable for the average practitioner (50\% level)}$$

Calculation of payment

Total number of adequate smears = 330
of which 240 done by GP or partner
          45 done by another GP
          30 done by DHA
          15 done privately

Therefore 285 were undertaken under General Medical Services.

$$\text{Maximum sum payable} \times \frac{285}{300} = \text{actual payment to each partner}$$

By April 1994 all FHSAs should have sufficient data on their computer systems to calculate entitlement to payments. Meanwhile, FHSAs may apportion tests of unclear origin in proportion to the known proportion of tests carried out by a GP for women on his or her list. For example, if the source of 12 tests is unclear and a GP has been responsible for taking the tests of 150 women on his or her eligible list of 192, then $\frac{150}{180} \times 12$, i.e. 10, of the unclear source tests will be allowed for payment.

An FHSA will also accept until 1994 information based on a GP's own records; GPs should use form FP/TCC to claim if the evidence from practice records indicates that a target has been reached. The validity of the claim may be checked by the FHSA.

Immunization for children aged two and under

A target payment system has replaced the previous individual payments for each immunization provided to children under the age of two.

Eligibility

A GP is eligible for a higher rate target payment if, on the first day of a quarter, the number of courses completed in each of the following groups of immunizations amounts on average to 90% of the number needed to achieve full immunization of all children aged two on his or her list. For the purpose of calculation, children aged two are defined as those born between the second day of the same quarter three years earlier and the first day of the corresponding quarter one year later, inclusive. For example, on 1 October 1993, the target population of children includes those born between 2 October 1990 and 1 October 1991.

Group one		Group two	Group three	
Diphtheria			Measles	1 dose
Tetanus	3 doses	Pertussis 3 doses	OR	
Poliomyelitis			Measles	
			Mumps	3 doses
			Rubella	

A GP will be eligible for a lower rate target payment if the average of courses completed amounts to 70% of the number needed for full immunization.

When the scheme was first proposed, payment was to be based on an individual GP's list; the scheme was subsequently modified so that target payments were calculated on a partnership basis.

Maximum sum payable

The maximum sum payable depends on the number of children aged two on the partnership list, compared with the average number.

The average number is calculated by multiplying 22 (the number of children aged two on the average GP's list) by the number of partners. The maximum sum payable is therefore:

$$\frac{\text{number of children aged two on partnership list}}{22 \times \text{number of partners}} \times \begin{array}{c} \text{maximum sum} \\ \text{payable to} \\ \text{average GP} \end{array}$$

Calculating the payment

The proportion of the payment due to the GP depends on the number of courses of immunization completed by doctors as part of general medical services as opposed to those completed elsewhere, for example at health authority clinics.

A course completed by other GPs (inside or outside the partnership) as part of general medical services will count towards the payment of the doctor making the claim. This means that if a child who has had all the completing doses moves and registers with another practice, the new practice can count that child towards its target payment even though it provided none of the immunizations.

A course will be considered as being completed by a GP as part of general medical services if he or she gives the final immunization needed to complete cover for the diseases in that group. Thus in group one the completing immunization will be the third poliomyelitis, if the child has also had three doses of diphtheria and tetanus vaccine.

Method of calculation

The first step is to decide how many completing immunizations are needed to reach a target. Twenty children have 60 immunization groups. So 42 completing immunizations would be required to reach the 70% target, and 54 for the 90% target. If the calculation results in a fraction, the target will be rounded to the nearest integer (0.5 being rounded down).

Secondly, it is necessary to decide whether a target has been reached by adding the numbers of completing immunizations carried out in each of the three groups. Thus, completing immunizations in excess of the target number in one group can top up the number in another group.

Thirdly, if a target has been achieved, it is necessary to calculate the maximum sum payable, comparing the actual number of eligible children with the average number.

Fourthly, it is necessary to count the number of completing immunizations carried out by GPs as part of general medical services for the three immunization groups, so that the appropriate proportion of the maximum sum payable can be calculated. Only one completing immunization per child can be counted for each group. Where the number of completing immunizations in each group done by GPs as part of general medical services is greater than the number of children needed to reach the target level, the latter figure is counted. For example, if a partnership has 40 children aged two on its list, 32 have completed their immunizations in each of the three groups, and all the completing doses were given by GPs, then the 70% target has been reached. As the 70% target number is 28 children who have had completing immunizations, only 28 count towards the work done by GPs in each group. Therefore, the number of completing immunizations done by GPs is regarded as $28 + 28 + 28 = 84$ ($= 100\%$ of the number needed to reach the 70% target).

Finally, the actual amount payable is then calculated by multiplying the maximum sum payable by the number of completing immunizations done as part of general medical services for the three groups added together, counted in the way described in the previous paragraph, and dividing by the number necessary to achieve the appropriate percentage cover. As there are three groups, the number necessary to achieve the target is the appropriate percentage of three times the number of children concerned.

If a GP works for another body such as a health authority, any immunization carried out as part of this other contract will not count towards payment. Work done by employed or attached staff at the direction of a GP as part of general medical services is however counted for payment.

How to claim

Claims should be made on form PT/TC1 no later than four months after the date to which the claim relates. GPs should report details of all immunizations to the appropriate health authorities and also inform the FHSA of any health authority appointments they hold which involve immunization work.

Example: six-partner practice

On the first day of the quarter a partnership of 6 doctors has 120 children aged two on its list. All 120 have had complete courses of immunizations against diphtheria, tetanus and poliomyelitis. Sixty of the completing immunizations were given by the GP's own practice, 30 by another GP practice and 30 by a DHA clinic.

Ninety of the children have had complete courses of immunization against pertussis. Of these 48 were given by the GP's own practice, none by another GP practice and 42 by a DHA clinic.

Seventy two of the children have been immunized against measles, mumps and rubella. Of these courses, 30 were given by the GP's own practice, 12 by another GP practice and 30 by a DHA clinic.

Step one: How many completing immunizations are needed to reach a target?

One hundred and twenty children have a maximum of 360 completing immunizations.
The 70% target requires 252 completing immunizations.
The 90% target requires 324 completing immunizations.

Step two: Has a target been reached?

Group 1 (DT and P)	120
Group 2 (Pertussis)	90
Group 3 (MMR)	72
Total	282

The 70% target has been reached.

Step three: What is the maximum sum payable?

$$\frac{120}{22 \times 6} \times \text{maximum sum payable to GP with an average list} = \text{maximum sum payable}$$

Step four: What proportion of the work needed to reach the target was done by GPs as part of general medical services?

Group 1	GP's own practice	60
	Another GP	30
	Total	90

but since 70% = 84 immunizations, this is treated as 84

Group 2	GP's own practice	48
	Another GP	0
	Total	48

Group 3	GP's own practice	30
	Another GP	12
	Total	42

	Group 1	84
	Group 2	48
	Group 3	42
	Total of completing doses regarded as carried out by GPs	174

Step five: How much is the payment?

Number of completing immunizations regarded as given by GPs = 174

Number of completing immunizations needed to reach 70%   = 252

Payment per partner $= \dfrac{174}{252} \times$ maximum sum payable for 70% target

Pre-school boosters for children aged five and under

Just as target payments have been introduced for immunization of children aged two and under, they are also paid for pre-school boosters for children aged five and under.

Eligibility

A GP is eligible for a target payment at the higher rate if, on the first day of each quarter, 90% of the children on the partnership list who are aged five have had reinforcing doses of diphtheria, tetanus and polio immunizations.

Children aged five are defined as those born between the second day of the same quarter six years earlier and the first day of the quarter a year later. For example, on 1 October 1993, the target population of children includes those born between 2 October 1987 and 1 October 1988.

If 70% of the children under five have reinforcing doses then a target payment at the lower rate will be made. The payment to be made will depend on the number of eligible patients, compared with the average number, and on the number of boosters given by GPs as opposed to those given by others. A child will only be considered as fully immunized if he or she has received booster doses of all three vaccines. One or two vaccines will not count.

Maximum sum payable

The number of children aged five on the partnership list compared to an average list will determine the maximum sum payable. The average number is calculated by multiplying 22 (the number of children aged five on the average GP's list) by the number of partners. The maximum sum payable is therefore:

$$\frac{\text{number of children aged 5 on the partnership list}}{22 \times \text{number of partners}} \times \frac{\text{maximum sum payable}}{\text{to average GP}}$$

Calculating the payment

The amount payable depends on the level of cover achieved and the number of complete booster doses of immunizations given by GPs as part of general medical services. Those provided by other sources, for example health authority clinics, do not count. Boosters given by other GPs under general medical services – for example if a child is given the necessary boosters by a GP in one practice and then moves to another part of the country and registers with a new doctor – will be counted in the target calculation of the claiming GP. The child will be counted towards the new GP's target levels and not those of the doctor who gave the boosters.

The first step in working out the payment to be made is to decide whether 90% or 70% of the total number of children have received booster doses for all three vaccines. In calculating the 90% or 70% target number, fractions will be rounded to the nearest integer (0.5 being rounded down). If a child does not have all three boosters at the same time, no account will be taken of them until all three boosters have been given. The booster will count as having been given by whoever gave the third booster dose.

Secondly, if a target is reached, the number of booster doses given as part of general medical services is counted so that the appropriate proportion of the maximum sum payable can be calculated.

Thirdly, the actual amount is calculated by multiplying the maximum sum payable by the number of booster doses given under general medical services, and dividing by the number of boosters necessary to achieve the appropriate percentage cover.

Work does not count as having been performed by a GP as part of general medical services if he or she immunizes children under a paid contract outside of general medical services. Work done by employed staff or attached staff under the direction of a GP as part of general medical services will however be counted.

How to claim

Claims should be made to the FHSA on form FP/TPB no later than four months after the date on which eligibility is assessed.

GPs are responsible for reporting all immunizations to the appropriate health authority as soon as they are given. This allows health authorities to provide GPs with information to help them in claiming payments.

GPs are also responsible for reporting to the FHSA any appointment that they hold with a health authority which includes providing pre-school boosters.

23 Vaccinations and immunizations

IN addition to the target payment system for the vaccination and immunization of children, a doctor who vaccinates a patient in accordance with public policy may claim a fee, provided the patient is on the GP's or a partner's list, or is eligible for treatment as a temporary resident, or is staying in the area for less than 24 hours.

If the vaccination is given by a suitably qualified person employed by the GP, or staff attached to the GP's practice and working under his or her direction, it is regarded as having been provided by the GP and the fee is payable.

Doctors who are paid to vaccinate patients by district or port health authorities cannot claim fees for vaccinations and immunizations.

Box 23.1: A vaccination fee is paid if:

- vaccination is in accordance with public policy
- patient is registered with the practice, a temporary resident, or staying in the area for less than 24 hours

---

In local outbreaks of disease emergency vaccination programmes are organized by health authorities. Any vaccination given by a doctor during an outbreak will qualify for payment if it is not given during a session in which the doctor is employed by the health authority, and if the person vaccinated is a member of a group for which vaccination has been recommended by the local specialist in public health medicine, or the person has been in close contact with a person suffering from the disease and the vaccination is subsequently approved by the public health medicine specialist, or the vaccination qualifies for an item-of-service payment in any case.

How to claim

Claims should be made on form FP73; both parts should be completed and sent to the FHSA, which will detach part 2 and send it to the health authority. Details of the diseases, the groups of persons affected for whom fees are payable and the fees are all set out in schedule 1 to paragraph 27 of the Red Book.

24 Supplying drugs and appliances

THERE are two ways in which GPs are paid for supplying drugs and appliances to patients:

- where these are supplied and personally administered to any patient by prescribing or dispensing doctors. This method is restricted to vaccines, anaesthetics, injections, diagnostic reagents, intrauterine devices, contraceptive caps and diaphragms, pessaries which are appliances, and sutures (including skin closure strips)
- where these are supplied by dispensing GPs to patients on their dispensing lists or to temporary residents in dispensing areas.

Payments for drugs and appliances include:

- the basic price less any discount calculated in accordance with the Red Book
- an on-cost allowance of a percentage of the basic price *before* deducting any discount
- a container allowance for each prescription
- a dispensing fee
- an allowance for VAT (payable only to GPs not registered for VAT)
- exceptional expenses as provided for in the Drug Tariff.

Payment for supplying oxygen and oxygen therapy equipment is calculated differently and is not subject to the discount arrangements.

A dispensing doctor who, with a patient's consent, issues a prescription form to enable him or her to obtain drugs or appliances from a pharmacist is not entitled to any remuneration under this part of the Red Book. If a practice provides evidence to the FHSA that because of its remoteness it cannot obtain any discount on the basic price of drugs and appliances, the FHSA may exempt the practice from the discount scale. An FHSA may grant exemption for up to one year, and this may be renewed if the practice is able to show that it is still experiencing difficulty in obtaining a discount.

If a practice can show that its remoteness or the small quantities of drugs and appliances it buys means that it obtains supplies at an average price at least 5% greater than the basic price, the FHSA can approve a special payment to remunerate the practice at a rate in excess of the basic drug price. Details are set out in paragraph 44.8 of the Red Book.

How to claim

Both dispensing and prescribing doctors should note, count and send all prescriptions with form FP34D to the Prescription Pricing Authority, no later than the fifth day of the month (for example, prescriptions relating to items supplied to patients during July should be sent by 5 August). GPs should ensure that prescriptions are endorsed in the appropriate column according to instructions in Red Book paragraph 44.9.

GPs in partnership should submit all prescriptions for pricing in one batch under the cover of one claim form for the partnership so that the appropriate discount rates may be applied. For calculation of the dispensing fee, doctors may if they wish subdivide the partnership batch into bundles relating to individual GPs, provided the bundles are joined together in one partnership batch.

Any doctor who wishes to examine his or her priced prescription forms should ask the FHSA to obtain these from the Prescription Pricing Authority.

Prescription charges

Items supplied by dispensing or prescribing doctors under the arrangements for personally administered items do not attract prescription charges and no charge should be made to the patient.

Practice accounts

To ensure the Inland Revenue's annual survey of doctors' practice expenses is accurate, GPs should show their actual expenditure on drugs and appliances (i.e. the amounts paid to their suppliers) as 'gross' in their accounts. Similarly, payments received for supplying drugs and appliances should be shown 'gross' as 'income' in the same way as other fees and allowances from the FHSA.

Oxygen therapy services

The Drug Tariff sets out the conditions for payment for the supply of oxygen and oxygen therapy equipment and applies to both pharmacists and dispensing doctors. The Red Book explains how dispensing doctors are paid for providing this service; they receive a fixed annual rental payable in monthly instalments for each oxygen set or stand they are authorized to hold by the FHSA, irrespective of whether the equipment is actually being used by a patient. Any dispensing doctor who wishes to hold oxygen equipment, or increase the number of sets or stands he or she is authorized to hold, should apply to the FHSA. The method of claiming and the rates of payment are described in paragraph 44, schedule 3 of the Red Book.

25 Teaching undergraduate medical students

GPs who assist a university department of general practice in the teaching of medical students by providing experience in general practice, will be paid according to the number of students involved and the time they spend in the practice.

The students should be from a recognized UK university department of general practice, which should arrange the training and confirm that it has taken place. If these conditions are met, a GP may claim a fee for each session a student is attached to the practice.

Time spent in the practice involves education and training in general medical services, including observing and learning about the work of the practice team.

A session consists of at least 2.5 hours in any 24 hour period; no more than two sessions per student per 24 hours may be claimed.

Only one GP may claim for any time spent by a student in a practice during any 24 hour period – normally the GP with whom the medical school arranged the attachment.

Box 25.1: Undergraduate medical students

- GPs may claim sessional fees for teaching undergraduate medical students
- each session consists of at least 2.5 hours of teaching activity
- no more than two sessions will be payable for each student in any 24 hour period

---

Claims should be made on form FP/UMS, setting out details of the number of sessions claimed and the time spent in the practice by each student. A GP should also send written confirmation from the university that students were attached to the practice at the times and dates on the claim form.

It is helpful to the FHSA if GPs specify which university department they are linked to for teaching undergraduate medical students.

26 The trainee practitioner scheme

Becoming a trainer

THE general practice sub-committee of the regional postgraduate education committee approves the appointment of trainers.

The sub-committee appoints a panel to interview the applicant and visits the practice before approving the appointment or reappointment of a trainer.

A GP will be approved as a trainer initially for a period not exceeding two years; this can be extended for periods of up to five years. If a trainer's practice circumstances change, the sub-committee may review, suspend, vary or terminate its approval.

If a GP applies to be a trainer and is dissatisfied with the decision of the sub-committee or is aggrieved by a decision affecting his or her appointment as a trainer, he or she may appeal to a national appeals committee within 28 days of receiving the sub-committee's decision. Details of how to appeal are set out in paragraphs 38.3 and 38.4 of the Red Book.

Conditions for payment

Any GP whose name is included in an FHSA's list and who has been approved as a trainer, is entitled to be paid while a trainee is working in the practice.

It is important that the trainer tells the FHSA when a new trainee appointment is made.

Training periods are normally for 12 months whole-time (or the equivalent part-time); this includes holidays (which should not exceed five weeks), public and bank holidays. Training may be divided between two practices: for example six months with one trainer and six months with another.

The trainer's grant cannot be paid for more than 12 months for the same trainee unless the training period is extended. If arrangements between the trainer and the trainee are terminated early, the sub-committee and FHSA should be told. There are certain circumstances in which a doctor may not need to undertake a full 12 month period of training; details are set out in paragraph 38.5(a) ii and iii of the Red Book.

If a trainer's appointment has less than a year to run, a new trainee should not be engaged without the approval of the sub-committee. A trainer is normally entitled to payment for only one trainee at a time, but payments for the salary of an additional trainee may be authorized if an overlap of training is approved by the regional postgraduate dean. An additional training grant is not paid in these circumstances.

A trainer must tell the FHSA and the sub-committee of any material changes in his or her practice circumstances, including a reduction in the amount of time any assistant works in the practice.

A GP should normally have a list of at least 2000 patients (or 1500 in rural areas) to be a trainer. Smaller lists may be approved by the sub-committee.

A trainer is responsible for appointing a trainee and should not pay a salary in excess of the amount approved by the FHSA. Trainees cannot be included in any medical list.

A doctor who has been appointed as a vocational scheme course organizer cannot also be paid a trainer's grant, even if he or she has a trainee in post.

Types of payment

A trainer receives these payments if a trainee is employed by the practice:

- a training grant
- reimbursement of the employer's share of the national insurance contributions paid for the trainee (The trainee pays the employee's share.)
- a motor vehicle allowance, according to vehicle type, if an additional vehicle is needed in the practice for the trainee
- the costs of installing an extra telephone extension at the surgery and a new telephone at the trainee's residence
- the rental charge for a telephone at the trainee's residence (provided the trainee is responsible for paying it) and the cost of installing and the rental charge for a bedroom telephone extension at the trainee's home, if the FHSA and trainer are both satisfied that it is necessary
- the trainee's salary which is related to the basic salary in his or her last regular NHS hospital post (Details of how this is calculated and of any increases applicable during the 12 month period are set out in paragraph 38.6(e) of the Red Book.)

  The FHSA will advise on how much should be paid, but it is essential that the FHSA is informed as soon as an appointment is made so that it can obtain information from the trainee's previous employer and determine without delay the salary to be paid.
- reimbursement of the trainee's medical defence organization subscription or premium costs, less the costs which would have been incurred if the trainee had taken out the basic subscription ('additional cover') payable by hospital doctors.

GP trainees' removal expenses

A doctor who moves from an NHS post to become a GP trainee (or moves from one training practice to another) and moves home as a result can claim removal expenses if the FHSA is satisfied that the removal is necessary. An FHSA may disregard any short unavoidable breaks in service due to unemployment or a locum appointment between leaving an NHS post and taking up the GP traineeship.

The payments are broadly similar to those made to hospital doctors under Section 26 of the NHS General Whitley Council Conditions of Service Handbook. Before incurring any expenditure, a trainee should ensure the FHSA agrees that the removal is necessary and expenses will be paid. The FHSA will examine the location of the trainer's practice area in relation to the trainee's existing home and the road links to the practice area.

The FHSA will also decide whether the proposed move is reasonable, that is to accommodation which is broadly comparable to that already occupied. If there is an obvious improvement in the standard of accommodation, the FHSA will relate payment of expenses to a notional purchase price or rent, assessed by a local estate agent and based on a property broadly comparable with the trainee's existing home, but related to prices in the new area. The FHSA will then make proportional payments towards the cost of purchase of property or rent in the new location, using the notional price or rent instead of the actual costs. The intention is that the move should cost the FHSA the same amount of money as if the trainee had moved to a house of identical standard. For instance, if a trainee leaves a two-bedroom semi-detached house which is sold for £50 000 and buys a four-bedroom house in the new area for £95 000, the FHSA may ask a local estate agent to assess the likely cost of the two-bedroom house in the new area. If the old property is assessed as being worth £65 000 in the new area, the FHSA will reduce the reimbursement of the costs involved in the purchase, such as solicitor's fees, by 30/95. If a trainee was compulsorily resident in health authority accommodation the FHSA has discretion to determine what is broadly comparable accommodation in the new area having regard to the standard of accommodation which the trainee may have had to accept in previous employment.

The Red Book conditions frequently refer to a householder, and define this as a trainee who occupied unfurnished accommodation of more than two main rooms, either rented or owner occupied, in the area of previous employment. The FHSA can ask the Secretary of State to vary this definition in cases of hardship.

Expenses of removal, house purchase and sale

Removal

Before the trainee moves his or her furniture and effects, the FHSA should approve the cost. If furniture is moved by contractors, three competitive tenders should be sent to the FHSA. A trainee may accept a tender other than the lowest, but the FHSA will base reimbursement on the lowest. Tenders should be subject to the usual conditions of removal and should not cover special services such as relaying carpets or taking down or putting up fixtures.

The expenditure reimbursed is the cost of moving furniture and effects belonging to the trainee and dependant members of his or her household from the old to the new home. This includes pedal cycles and heavy but ordinary items of gardening equipment or furniture, but not items such as grand pianos which require special arrangements. Livestock apart from domestic pets must be conveyed at the trainee's own expense.

The cost of moving from the old home into storage and then on to the new home can also be reimbursed. If housing difficulties make it necessary, payment will be made of the cost of moving some articles such as cots, perambulators, radio, television and high-fidelity equipment into temporary accommodation in furnished rooms while moving the majority of furniture into storage.

Storage

If furniture and effects have to be put into storage, the cost will be reimbursed. If a trainee cannot find suitable accommodation and has to store furniture while occupying temporary unfurnished accommodation in the new area, he or she will only be reimbursed storage charges if the rent in the new area exceeds that in the old; otherwise payment will be restricted to the amount by which the new rent plus the storage charges exceeds the old rent.

Insurance on furniture in transit will be allowed up to the value for which it is normally insured. Extra insurance charges on stored furniture will be treated as part of storage charges.

Legal and estate agent fees

A householder may claim reimbursement for all reasonable legal and other expenses (including VAT) if a house is purchased because of the traineeship and is the first permanent unfurnished accommodation occupied in the area of the training practice, or a house is sold immediately before taking up the traineeship. The removal must be for more than six months and receipts and vouchers to prove expenditure must be produced. FHSAs like to have estate agents' details of the properties that are being bought and sold, if estate agents have been used. Expenses related to house purchase include solicitors' fees, stamp duty, land registration fees, incidental legal expenses, expenses in connection with a mortgage or loan including guarantee and survey fees, and the costs of a private survey, an electrical wiring test and a drains test. If a trainee incurs expenses relating to a proposed purchase which is subsequently abandoned, the FHSA may reimburse these if they are reasonable relative to the work done. The FHSA needs to be satisfied that the trainee was not responsible for abandoning the purchase and that abandonment was reasonable.

Expenses related to house sale include solicitors' fees, legal expenses incurred in mortgage redemption, and house agents' or auctioneers' fees. If a trainee sells a house without using an estate agent, incidental expenses may be claimed up to a set limit to cover telephone calls, advertising and postage.

No compensation can be paid for any loss on the sale of a house consequent on taking up a traineeship.

If a trainee lets the house instead of selling it, legal expenses relating to letting may be reimbursed, but legal expenses in connection with a subsequent sale will not then be reimbursed.

A trainee who obtains a bridging loan will be reimbursed interest charges (net after tax relief); these will be for a loan not exceeding the estimated selling price of the old house and may continue for up to three months if the FHSA is satisfied that the trainee acted reasonably in buying a house before selling the old house. Bridging loan interest reimbursement may continue beyond three months if the FHSA is convinced that the trainee is making every effort to sell the old home at a reasonable figure.

Tenancy

Within a defined limit, the costs of a tenancy agreement, house agents' fees and a drains test can be reimbursed to a trainee who rents furnished accommodation. These expenses are not reimbursed to trainees who move into rented lodgings.

Travelling expenses

Preliminary visit

A trainee may claim travelling and subsistence expenses for visiting the new area of traineeship to search for accommodation. These are paid at the same rate as those payable for educational courses; the subsistence element will not be paid for more than four nights. A trainee who takes his or her spouse receives additional subsistence for the same period at two-thirds of the rate paid to the trainee. Any children aged 12 years or over accompanying the trainee will attract a subsistence payment of two-thirds, and any child under 12 years of half the trainee's rate.

Journey from the old home to the new

The cost of one journey (and if the length of journey warrants it, subsistence allowance) will be paid for the trainee and dependants; the dependants will include anyone under 21 years moving to the new home with the trainee even though that person may be earning his or her own living. The term dependant also includes one servant or nurse.

Return visit to superintend the removal

Travelling expenses will be paid if a trainee returns home to superintend the removal. Subsistence allowances may also be paid if the number of nights, when added to the period of the preliminary visit, does not exceed four. Subsistence is not paid if the trainee uses or could use the old accommodation or stays with relatives.

Season tickets

A trainee may claim for the unexpired value of a railway or bus season ticket if the amount is irrecoverable from the railway or bus company. Reimbursement will relate only to the quarter current at the time of removal.

Losses arising from educational commitments

Details of the amounts and conditions relating to claims for losses arising from educational arrangements are set out in paragraph 38.17(b) of the Red Book. An allowance may be claimed if the move results in a loss of school fees paid in the old area, or towards the lodging costs of a child who has to be left in the old area for educational reasons.

Allowance during search for accommodation

Subsistence

A married trainee (or a single trainee with equivalent responsibilities) who does not find suitable accommodation before taking up the traineeship and leaves the family at home, may claim night subsistence equivalent to that payable for training courses. This amount will be paid if the FHSA is satisfied that the trainee is making every effort to find suitable family accommodation.

Visits home

Subsistence allowances will continue even if the trainee returns home to the old area at weekends provided he or she is away from lodgings for no more than three nights. Travelling expenses will be reimbursed weekly for visits home.

Excess daily travel

A trainee who is able to travel daily to the area of the traineeship whilst looking for suitable family accommodation may be reimbursed the extra cost of travelling by bus, second class rail or private motor vehicle. This cannot exceed the long-term subsistence rate and will continue only if the FHSA is satisfied that the trainee is actively seeking suitable family accommodation.

Miscellaneous expenses grant

A miscellaneous removals expenses grant (set out in paragraph 43 of Section 26 of the General Whitley Council Conditions of Service Handbook) is paid to a trainee to compensate for the additional expenses of occupying new permanent accommodation. The amount is paid in full to trainees who have not made a similar claim during the previous two years. The expenses of a trainee who has made a similar claim will be limited to the actual expenditure incurred, and reimbursement will be conditional on submitting a statement of expenditure to the FHSA. Paragraph 38.16(c) of the Red Book gives some examples of expenditure that would qualify, such as installing a television aerial, plumbing in a washing machine and redirecting of mail.

Continuing commitments allowance

If a trainee incurs rent and rates expenditure in the new area whilst incurring similar expenditure in the old area, an allowance will be paid to offset the costs.

- Married trainees or those with equivalent domestic commitments will be paid an allowance equal to the continuing commitments in the old area or the long-term night subsistence allowance, whichever is the less, for up to three months from the date the family join the trainee in the new area.
- Single householders will be paid a similar allowance for up to three months from the date of taking up the traineeship.
- Single trainees will be paid whichever is the less of the continuing commitment in the old area, or the retention of rooms allowance set out in paragraph 38.11, for a period of up to three months from taking up the traineeship.

If any part of the accommodation in the old area is let, the rent received will be deducted from any amount payable. The allowance will not be paid when a trainee is receiving bridging loan expenses as set out in paragraph 38.13(a).

Retention of rooms allowance

If a trainee is temporarily absent from lodgings in the area of the traineeship (for instance at weekends) but has to pay to retain the accommodation, he or she will be able to claim an allowance unless a night subsistence allowance for weekend periods of absence is being paid.

Payment of rent of unoccupied property

If a trainee has to commence payment of rent on a property in the new area while still paying rent in the old area, he or she may be reimbursed up to the amount of the long-term night subsistence rate.

Payment of travelling expenses and additional accommodation costs in lieu of removal expenses

If a trainee establishes a permanent home in order to undertake his or her vocational training and chooses to travel from home to the location of the various posts he or she holds during the training period rather than move, excess daily travelling expenses can be claimed. For example, if the trainee lives three miles from a hospital where he or she holds a hospital post and chooses to travel 23 miles when he or she moves into general practice, the trainee will be entitled to claim for 20 miles per journey by way of excess travelling, if the FHSA is satisfied that removal expenses would have been appropriate had the trainee chosen to move.

A trainee may choose to take temporary lodgings away from his or her permanent home and close to the training practice, in which case actual expenses may be paid.

Payment of expenses of trainees when on call

A trainee who qualifies to receive payments under the above two paragraphs and is required by the practice to be on call may stay in lodgings close to the practice on those nights and weekends when on call. On such occasions, the trainee will not qualify for excess daily travelling but will receive reimbursement of the actual lodging expenses, limited to the long-term night subsistence rate.

Excess rent allowance

The arrangements for excess rent allowance are described in Section 26 of the General Whitley Council Conditions of Service Handbook. This allowance compensates a trainee who moves to a more expensive area to take up a traineeship and relates to either owner-occupied or rented accommodation. Full details of the scheme are set out in paragraphs 38.19 to 38.22 of the Red Book. Trainees should obtain advice from FHSAs about the complex payment arrangements.

Interview expenses

A trainee attending a selection interview with a trainer is paid travelling and subsistence expenses unless the application is withdrawn or the offer of appointment is declined.

Payments to trainees during sickness

If a trainee is sick and absent from the practice for up to two weeks, payments to the trainer will continue, but will be abated by any statutory sick pay (SSP) received. It will not usually be necessary to extend the traineeship in those circumstances. If a trainee is absent for more than two weeks, the national insurance contributions and the salary of the trainee will continue to be reimbursed for up to three months; this will again be abated by SSP, or when SSP ceases by any sickness or injury benefits payable under the National Insurance Acts. Payment of the training grant and car allowance will cease during sickness. The Secretary of State has discretion to extend payments for absences beyond three months and application should be made to the FHSA. The traineeship may be extended to allow training to be completed. Trainers should tell the FHSA when their trainee is unable to work because of sickness.

Maternity leave for trainees

Payment of the trainee's salary will continue to be made during maternity leave taken, subject to the conditions in paragraphs 38.28 to 38.42 of the Red Book.

Payments of expenses involved in sitting examinations for postgraduate qualifications

A trainee who sits an examination for a postgraduate qualification may be paid travelling and subsistence allowances at the rates paid for approved educational activities. No claim can be made for an examination fee or the cost of typing or binding papers for the examining body. The trainee should send form GPCF3 to the FHSA, with confirmation by the trainer that the trainee attended the examination.

27 The doctors' retainer scheme

THIS scheme is for doctors working not more than one day a week who wish to remain in touch with medicine so that they can return to a fuller commitment to the NHS when circumstances permit. They can do a small amount of specially arranged paid professional work, attend postgraduate medical education sessions, and receive a small retainer to help meet their expenses. The scheme is primarily intended to help women doctors, but it also applies to men. It is administered by Regional Health Authorities and clinical tutors working under the direction of postgraduate deans and regional postgraduate medical committees.

The scheme requires a doctor to work at least one half-day per month and to be prepared to take on sessional work up to a maximum of one day per week, provided this does not conflict with family commitments. These sessions may be in a practice approved by the regional postgraduate education committee where the doctor works as an assistant. The time worked is to be agreed by the doctor, the practice and the clinical tutor, and the terms of employment are to be agreed by the doctor and the practice.

The FHSA reimburses a practice which employs a retainer scheme doctor up to a maximum of the fee for a notional half-day per week. A notional half-day is defined as 3.5 hours, and subject to the maximum of one half-day per week, a practice can agree with the FHSA how many sessions are claimed.

Box 27.1: Doctors' retainer scheme

the FHSA pays the employing practice for a maximum of one notional half-day per week

---

Information about the scheme can be obtained from regional advisers in general practice.

28 Postgraduate education allowance

Who is eligible?

A practitioner is paid an allowance if he or she:

- has attended 25 days of accredited postgraduate education spread reasonably over the five years preceding the claim
- has during that time attended at least two accredited courses in each of these three subject areas:

  health promotion and illness prevention
  disease management
  service management.

Each doctor in a job-sharing arrangement is eligible for the allowance if he or she individually satisfies the criteria.

Which courses qualify?

Courses are accredited if approved by the regional adviser on postgraduate education in England, or by the postgraduate dean in consultation with the associate adviser in Wales. Anyone planning a course should apply for approval. The regional adviser or postgraduate dean will accredit the course, and determine its duration and the subject areas of its sessions. The three subject areas mentioned above cover the following:

'Health promotion and the prevention of illness' includes promoting healthy living and preventing disease, injury and ill health.

'Disease management' includes the natural history of disease and injury and treatment and care of the sick and terminally ill.

'Service management' includes aspects of providing efficient care to patients including data and record systems, the use of technology and of staff and health care teams, practice organization, cost effective prescribing, quality assurance and audit, and the interface between different caring services.

A course may be formal or informal – for example at a GP's surgery – and may run continuously for a specific period or comprise separate sessions held regularly and frequently in a single subject area.

Distance learning

Distance learning packages may be accredited by the regional adviser, who will specify a notional length in qualifying half-days.

Unpaid clinical attachments

Unpaid clinical attachments supervised by a consultant and (normally) supernumerary to establishment may be accredited. In these cases the regional adviser will specify its subject area and its notional length in qualifying half-days.

Doctors teaching on courses

A doctor teaching at an accredited course will be considered to have attended that course for half a day. If the course lasts for a longer period and the doctor attends the full course, he or she will be credited with the same attendance as other GPs. If the doctor teaches during sessions covering more than half a day in total, he or she will be considered as having attended those sessions.

Doctors becoming GPs for the first time more than 12 months after completing vocational training

A doctor joining the list more than 12 months after completing vocational training will be paid the full allowance if the following conditions are satisfied:

- the first claim is within 12 months of becoming a GP
- each subsequent claim is made within 15 months of the preceding claim
- **first claim:** the doctor has attended at least five days of accredited postgraduate educational courses within the year preceding the claim;
  second claim: the doctor has attended at least 10 days of accredited postgraduate education in the two years preceding the claim, including at least one accredited course in each of two subject areas;
  third claim: the doctor has attended at least 15 days of accredited postgraduate education courses reasonably spread over the three years preceding the claim, including at least one accredited course in each of the three subject areas;
  fourth claim: the doctor has attended at least 20 days of accredited postgraduate education courses spread reasonably across the four years preceding the claim, including at least one accredited course in each of the three subject areas.

Doctors becoming GPs for the first time within 12 months of completing vocational training

A doctor will be paid the full allowance for the four quarters preceding the claim provided the first claim is made within 12 months of completing vocational training.

Subsequently, provided each claim is made within 15 months of the preceding claim, the doctor will be paid the full allowance if the following conditions are met:

second-first subsequent-claim: the doctor has attended at least five days of accredited postgraduate education courses during the year preceding the claim;

third claim: the doctor has attended at least 10 days of accredited postgraduate education courses in the two years preceding the claim, including at least one accredited course in each of two subject areas;

fourth claim: the doctor has attended at least 15 days of accredited postgraduate education courses over the three years preceding the claim, including at least one accredited course in each of the three subject areas;

fifth claim: the doctor has attended at least 20 days of accredited postgraduate education courses over the four years preceding the claim, including at least one accredited course in each of the three subject areas.

What happens if a GP fails to maintain the five year programme?

If a GP is unable to qualify for the full allowance, he or she will be eligible to claim a reduced allowance if the following conditions are met:

Level 1 can be claimed if a doctor has attended at least five days of accredited postgraduate education courses in the five years preceding the claim.

Level 2 can be claimed if a doctor has attended at least 10 days of accredited postgraduate education courses in the five years preceding the claim, including at least one accredited course in each of two subject areas.

Level 3 can be claimed if a doctor has attended at least 15 days of accredited postgraduate education courses over the five years preceding the claim, including at least one accredited course in each of the three subject areas.

Level 4 can be claimed if a doctor has attended at least 20 days of accredited postgraduate education courses over the five years preceding the claim, including at least one accredited course in each of the three subject areas.

Claims

Form FP/PEA is used to claim payment. Claims can be made at any date following the completion of courses, and the allowance will be paid for the following 12 month period. No new claim can normally be made within 12 months of the date of the previous claim. The FHSA will require documentary proof of attendance.

It should be noted that an FHSA may withhold all or part of an allowance if it considers that a course has been unreasonably repeated, or that the days are spread unreasonably between years. A GP is not expected to claim for more than 10 days in any year.

Arrangements after 1990

Doctors were eligible for the full allowance if by April 1990 they had attended five days of accredited education in the preceding year.

If they did not satisfy this requirement, they could still claim the allowance by 1 October 1990 if they had completed five days of accredited education in the period from 1 April 1989, and were considered to have been eligible for the allowance on 1 April 1990. They could make the next claim after 1 April 1991.

Doctors who qualified for the full allowance were and will be eligible for full payment in subsequent years provided the following criteria were met:

- each **subsequent claim** was made within 15 months of the preceding claim
- **second claim** (after 1 April 1991): the doctor had attended at least 10 days of accredited postgraduate education courses in the two years preceding the claim including at least one course in each of two of the subject areas;
- **third claim**: the doctor had attended at least 15 days of accredited postgraduate courses spread over the three years preceding the claim, including at least one accredited course in each of the three subject areas;
- **fourth claim**: the doctor had attended at least 20 days of accredited postgraduate education course spread over four years preceding the claim, including at least one accredited course in each of the three subject areas.

Courses held between 1 April 1989 and 31 March 1990 were considered as accredited if they were:

- approved under Section 63; or
- an individual clinical attachment, under consultant supervision and normally supernumerary to establishment.

The regional adviser determined the length and subject group of such courses and advised the FHSA.

29 Reimbursing rent and rates

Who is eligible?

ANY GP with at least 100 patients is eligible, but a lower list size may be accepted by the FHSA if it is being built up.

Acceptance of premises

Purpose of the scheme

The scheme reimburses GPs the cost of rent and rates on practice accommodation by taking account of what each doctor actually pays or may be deemed to have paid.

GPs who purpose-build or substantially alter their surgery accommodation may be reimbursed a cost rent. (This scheme is explained on pages 134–144.)

Because the scheme reduces significantly an individual GP's personal financial interest in the expense incurred, an FHSA must satisfy itself that premises are being used effectively and that any expansion of premises is in the interests of the NHS.

Moving premises

Because the FHSA must ensure that a doctor's premises and their use are reasonable, it also has to assess a proposed move in the same terms. If a move or proposed expansion of premises unreasonably increases costs under the scheme without improving services to NHS patients, an FHSA will not increase reimbursement beyond that already being paid. For example, the FHSA, LMC and district health authority may have decided a health centre should be provided in a new housing development; in these circumstances the FHSA would be unlikely to agree to new practice premises in the same area being reimbursed under the scheme. Similarly, a practice may want to leave a health centre and provide its own surgery premises; unless the FHSA is satisfied there are good reasons for doing so, it will not increase reimbursement beyond that already being paid for the health centre.

New branch surgeries

Payments for new branch surgeries are limited to the size of accommodation which the FHSA regards as reasonable for NHS patients in the area, and the

FHSA will also need to be satisfied that the population in the area is best served by the proposed new consultation facilities.

Consulting the FHSA before changing surgery accommodation

Since payments are only made if the accommodation is accepted by the FHSA, a practice must consult it before changing its premises; otherwise:

- the FHSA may not agree that the changes improve services to patients
- the GP may not receive an increased notional rent or may be unaware of other ways in which improvements to premises can be funded.

What should doctors do if they are unhappy with an FHSA decision about their surgery premises?

If a practice disagrees with an FHSA's decision on accepting its current or proposed premises or proposed enlargements for reimbursement under the scheme, it should appeal to the Secretary of State for Health within two months of the decision, explaining why it is dissatisfied.

What is an FHSA looking for when approving premises under the scheme?

The scheme applies to premises included in the medical list where GPs see NHS patients at advertised open surgery sessions and by appointment. The FHSA has to be satified that reasonable use is made of the premises; *any premises used for only occasional consultations will not be accepted.*

Premises may be either a separate unit or part of a residence, and either rented or owned by a GP or a close relative of the GP. (The definition of close relative includes a spouse, child, sibling, parent or grandparent of the doctor or his or her spouse.) Premises owned or rented by a close relative are treated as if they were owned or rented by the GP.

Only those parts of the premises used directly for NHS practice will be accepted for payment; for example, garages and carports are acceptable only if they form part of separate practice premises. Parking space for GPs used by both the practice and patients is acceptable.

Residential accommodation is not accepted for payment unless occupied by someone (other than a GP) who answers patients' calls after surgery hours; any rent received from the occupant will be taken into account in assessing the level of payment.

If the surgery accommodation is rented, or is included within premises subject to a rental agreement, the FHSA may wish to see the lease or tenancy agreement. The GP will need to state whether he or she or a member of his or her family is related to or in any way connected with the lessor, including a private company of which he or she or any of his or her partners or a member of his or her or their families is a member.

Apart from certain premises in rural areas, main or branch surgery accommodation will not be approved for the scheme unless the FHSA, following a visit, is satisfied that the following criteria are met:

- ease of access to premises and movement within them, bearing in mind the needs of the elderly, the disabled (including those in wheelchairs) and mothers with young children
- provision of properly equipped treatment and consulting rooms, with adequate arrangements to ensure the privacy of consultations and of patients when dressing or undressing, either in a separate examination room or in a screened off area around an examination couch within the consulting or treatment room
- convenient access for the GP, staff and patients (including wheelchair access) to adequate lavatory and washing facilities (GPs should have a wash basin in or immediately adjacent to their consulting room.)
- adequate internal waiting areas with enough seating for normal requirements, and provision (either in the reception area or elsewhere) for patients to communicate confidentially with reception staff, including by telephone
- premises, fittings and furniture to be kept clean and in good repair, with adequate standards of lighting, heating and ventilation
- adequate fire precautions, including provision for safe exit from the premises, designed according to the building regulations agreed with the local fire authority
- adequate security for records, prescription pads, pads of doctors' statements, and drugs
- if minor surgery is undertaken, a suitable room and equipment for this purpose.

In some rural areas GPs consult in premises normally used for other purposes (e.g. village halls, public houses). These cannot be expected to satisfy all the above criteria; however, the consulting facilities must be adequate.

FHSAs routinely visit premises and if a surgery does not comply with these standards, they may abate or withhold rent and rates reimbursement; six months' notice must be given before taking this action and GPs can appeal to the Secretary of State against their decision.

FHSAs may also ask medical service committees to investigate the acceptability of a GP's surgery accommodation under paragraph 27 of the terms of service.

How payments are made

FHSAs calculate rent and rates reimbursements as follows.

Rents

- cost rents for new separate purpose-built accommodation or its equivalent (*see* pages 134–144)
- notional rents for owner-occupiers, for separate premises or premises forming part of a residence
- payments for rented separate premises, for premises in rented residences or for premises rented from local authorities which charge an economic rent.

How are notional rents and payments for rented premises decided?

Notional rents and payments for rented premises are decided after the current market rent has been assessed by the district valuer.

What is the current market rent?

Current market rent is the amount that the district valuer considers might reasonably be expected to be paid for the premises at the time of valuation.

Rates

- uniform business rates
- water rates
- sewerage, miscellaneous, environmental, drainage or embankment rates.

Rates will not be reimbursed separately if already included in the rent.

Water meters

Water companies may offer GPs the option of paying for water on a metered basis instead of through a charge calculated on the rateable value of the premises. The NHS should benefit from any savings achieved by moving to a metered supply and FHSAs encourage doctors to do so if savings are possible.

If it can be shown that changing to a metered system may produce savings in comparison with water rates, and that the annual savings may be sufficient to cover within four years the historic cost of installing a water meter, installation costs and meter charges will be directly reimbursed irrespective of whether the expected savings are actually achieved. Water companies will advise GPs of the likely costs involved.

Refuse collection charges

If a local authority levies a separate charge for collecting trade refuse from surgeries, or health authorities or private contractors make alternative arrangements for which they charge, the lowest charge levied may be reimbursed if receipts are submitted.

Box 29.1: Rent and rates scheme: types of direct reimbursement

- cost rents
- notional rents
- rental reimbursements
- uniform business rates
- water rates
- sewerage rates etc.
- water meter installation costs and charges
- refuse collection charges

Why are payments abated?

Abatement because of private income

If a doctor earns private income from work undertaken at surgery premises accepted under the scheme, payments will be reduced if gross income from this work is at least 10% of total gross income. Private income includes all professional income received from other than public sources. A reduction of 10% is made if between 10% and 20% of gross income is from private work, of 20% if between 20% and 30% is, and so on.

A GP undertaking private work at a surgery not within the scheme may have reimbursement on his or her NHS surgery reduced unless it can be shown that the private income is wholly derived from work at the private surgery. Practice accounts should identify this income separately.

Abatement because surgery accommodation is used by other bodies

If the surgery accommodation is used by a DHA or some other organization, payments will be reduced by the amount of rent received from that source.

Separate premises

Separate premises are defined as self-contained premises used only for practice purposes and assessed separately for rates.

Payment for rented premises will be the lease rent or the district valuer's assessment of current market rent, whichever is lower.

In all cases where the rent covers non-practice accommodation, the current market rent will be assessed on the basis described in the Red Book.

If the GP owns the freehold of separate premises or the premises are held under a ground lease by the GP, a notional rent is assessed by the district valuer at the date of occupation.

If rates are not included in the rent paid under a lease or tenancy agreement, or general rates are paid for premises owned by the GP, these are reimbursed separately. They will be abated according to the division of gross value for rating purposes, as assessed by the district valuer, if non-practice accommodation is included in the premises.

Practice accommodation in a residence

If the accommodation is in a residence owned by the doctor, notional rent and rates payments are only made for that part used regularly and substantially for practice purposes. If a room is used for both domestic and practice purposes a part payment is made. For example, a room used regularly for a certain number of hours a day as a waiting area for patients will be accepted for partial payment under the scheme as accommodation in dual use. However, if only minimal domestic use is made of some part of the accommodation, it will be accepted as wholly used for practice purposes.

If a branch surgery is in a private residence and advertised surgery sessions are held on less than three days a week, an FHSA will not accept any of the accommodation as being in dual use and thereby eligible for partial payment under the scheme.

FHSAs determine notional rent for surgeries on the advice of district valuers who assess current market rental value of that part of the premises used for practice purposes.

The gross rateable value of the residence as a whole will be apportioned by the district valuer according to the accommodation provided by the GP for practice purposes and agreed by the FHSA. For those parts of the accommodation in dual use, payment will be based on the ratio between the apportioned value of the parts used solely for practice and non-practice purposes. Thus, in the case of a residence with a gross rateable value of £360, where the district valuer advises that £200 relates to accommodation in sole use for non-practice purposes and £100 to sole use for practice purposes – a ratio of 2 to 1 – the apportioned gross value for rating the remaining part in dual use would be $£(1/3 \times 60) = £20$.

If the practice accommodation is part of a residence rented by the GP, payments under the scheme relate solely to that part used regularly for practice purposes. The rental value and gross value for rating will be apportioned by the district valuer as described above, in order to calculate the rent and rates payments due under the scheme.

Claims for payment and accounting procedures

GPs should ensure that they actually claim reimbursement of rents paid and of rates and water rates. FHSAs can provide many examples of practices which never claim or claim only irregularly!

Rent

Claims should be sent to the 'responsible' FHSA. Most FHSAs automatically pay monthly, rather than quarterly in arrears, unless requested not to do so. Monthly advances will not be made if the rent is paid at greater than monthly intervals, but reimbursement will be made as soon as possible after receipts are submitted.

Rates

Rates will be reimbursed as soon as possible after receipts are sent to the FHSA. Claims on form PREM2 should be sent to the FHSA each year, within seven days of 30 June.

Details of practice accommodation

When a GP acquires premises, form PREM1 must be completed in triplicate giving details of the accommodation; two copies are sent to the FHSA and one is retained by the GP. Form PREM1 must also be sent to the FHSA whenever accommodation or ownership changes. As soon as form PREM1 is received, the FHSA will tell the GP whether the premises are accepted under the scheme. If the accommodation forms part of a residence, the FHSA will also confirm whether the schedule of accommodation used for practice purposes is acceptable.

A GP will be told what payment will be made by the FHSA as soon as it has received the district valuer's opinion.

An FHSA officer (together with an LMC representative) may need to visit the premises before the FHSA gives its approval. Almost always, the district valuer will also need to visit the practice.

What should a GP do if dissatisfied with the payment proposed by the FHSA?

If a practice is not satisfied with the proposed payment or with the apportionment of the gross rateable value where non-practice accommodation is involved, it may submit independent evidence to the FHSA for the district valuer to consider. If the practice is still dissatisfied, it may appeal to the Secretary of State.

Declaring rent and rates expenses to the Inland Revenue

To avoid confusion in the Inland Revenue's annual survey of practice expenses, all GPs should ensure that their rent and rates expenses are shown as gross expenditure in their accounts and direct reimbursements under the scheme are shown as income alongside other forms of income from the FHSA.

Review of payments

Notional rents

The notional rent is reviewed three yearly after the date of any assessment made on or after 1 October 1976.

When a review is due, the FHSA will send form PREM1 to the GP some time before the review date. The form should be completed and returned to the FHSA, which will then send it to the district valuer so that any change in valuation can be reflected in increased payments, as close as possible to the review date. Although it is in their interest to return the form to the FHSA as soon as possible some GPs fail to do so and others do so only after a considerable delay.

A minor change in the accommodation may be accepted by the FHSA, but a significant change normally requires an FHSA officer to visit the surgery. The district valuer may also make a visit, particularly if the practice accommodation forms part of a residence and there has been a change in the ratio of domestic to practice use.

The district valuer may be prepared to negotiate with GPs or their professional advisers in order to agree a current market rent or the apportionment to be recommended to the FHSA.

GPs are notified by the FHSA of the revised level of payment, which normally continues for three years unless there are changes to the premises.

Accommodation in a residence owned by a doctor

The notional rent is reviewed every three years in the same way as for separate premises.

Rented premises

The assessment of the current market rent of accommodation rented by a GP is related to the period of the lease or rental agreement and is reviewed whenever the lease or agreement is changed.

Review of rating assessments

Whenever the rating assessment changes, the apportionment of the gross value used to calculate the reimbursement of rates and rent (or notional rent) of surgeries in residences is also reviewed.

GPs should tell FHSAs when their rating assessments change so that the apportionment can be reviewed. If a practice is dissatisfied with a revised apportionment, it can appeal to the Secretary of State.

Local authority economic rents

This part of the rent and rates scheme allows an FHSA to reimburse an 'economic rent' charged by a local authority for practice premises.

Circular LASSL 80(3) (or in Wales, WO 38/80), which is available from FHSAs, defines 'economic rent', explains how it is calculated and describes the certification necessary for payment.

The premises must be accepted by the FHSA and the abatement for private practice may apply.

If a practice is provided with temporary accommodation by a local authority, it may be charged for restoring it to some other use, such as housing. These costs should not be included in the rent, but the FHSA should be told of any liability for such charges as soon as the premises are occupied, because the practice may be eligible for help in meeting them. A claim may be met in full if the FHSA is satisfied that:

- the work is necessary to restore the surgery to its intended future use
- the cost is not excessive
- the practice's use of the premises was not unreasonably short.

30 Improving surgery premises

THERE are three main sources of financial help for improving premises:

- notional rent reimbursement
- improvement grants
- cost rent payments.

Notional rent reimbursement

Minor improvements to premises that do not qualify for an improvement grant or a cost rent payment normally justify an increased notional rent.

Improvement grants

These grants may be available to fund improvements. The FHSA's prior approval must be obtained, and because an FHSA has to take account of its existing priorities and cash allocation, applications will not always be approved.

GPs may be eligible for grants of between one-third and two-thirds of the cost of improving their surgeries, including professional fees associated with the design and supervision of the work, and statutory fees charged by a local authority for approving plans and inspecting the building.

Grants are not available for projects costing less than the figure in schedule 2 of the improvement grant section of the Red Book.

Who is eligible?

All GPs providing unrestricted general medical services are eligible if their NHS list (or average list in a partnership) includes at least 500 patients in urban areas or 350 in rural areas, or is expected to reach these levels within a year.

Which projects are eligible?

Projects which qualify include:

- adding a new room: for example a consulting room, a room for minor surgery, patients' toilet and washing facilities
- bringing into use a room not previously used

- enlarging an existing room
- improving the heating system
- extending telephone facilities
- double-glazing
- installing a security system
- installing fire precautions
- car and pram parking
- improving access to the premises, including wheelchair access.

The work must significantly improve existing arrangements. When making its assessment the FHSA takes account of its standards for surgery accommodation.

The work must improve what already exists, rather than create new premises. Thus, the premises to be improved must normally be in current use for NHS practice and must already be covered by the rent and rates scheme.

However, premises not previously used for NHS purposes may be eligible if the FHSA considers they could have been used for NHS practice in their existing state. In such circumstances, the grant cannot exceed a specified maximum.

GPs must have security of tenure: the premises should be owned by the practice or held on a lease at least as long as the minimum period of use specified in the scheme. If premises are leased, the FHSA must be sent the landlord's written approval of the alteration.

If work is undertaken on premises not used solely for NHS practice, a grant will be paid only for the practice part of the accommodation.

If it is intended to extend existing premises a grant is only paid if:

- any building separate from the main building is attached by at least a covered passageway
- the total area of the accommodation in the completed project does not exceed that specified in the cost rent schedules (*see* pages 139–140).

Which projects are ineligible?

The improvement grant scheme will not cover:

- *any project where a contract has been entered into, or work commenced, without the FHSA's prior approval*
- *any expenses on which a tax allowance is being claimed* (*see* page 133)
- the initial provision of premises including the costs of acquiring land, existing buildings or new buildings
- the replacement or part replacement of premises: including projects such as building an extension to accommodate part or all of the practice premises so that the original premises can revert to private use
- the provision or replacement of furniture (except if it is built-in), furnishings, floor covering or equipment

- the repair or maintenance of premises, furniture, furnishings, floor covering and equipment
- the restoration of structural damage or deterioration
- any work connected with the domestic part of the accommodation
- that part of an extension which, when added to the original practice accommodation remaining in use after the new work has been completed, exceeds the area allowed under the cost rent schedules
- any extension not attached to the main building by at least a covered passageway.

Apportioning total cost if premises are used for other purposes

If a project includes expenditure not attributable to NHS general practice, costs must be divided. Apportionment may also be necessary if the premises are used for a substantial amount of private practice.

Guarantee of continued use after improvement

Before a grant is paid, GPs have to give an undertaking that the premises will continue to be used for NHS practice for the minimum period specified in the scheme and that they are willing to repay a proportion of the grant if this undertaking is broken.

How to apply for a grant

GPs should obtain advice from the FHSA and its medical adviser at an early stage, to avoid unnecessary design work and expense.

An application form should be sent to the FHSA, with the following documentation:

- estimate of total costs, including fees, prepared by a builder, architect, surveyor or other qualified person
- sketch plan of the existing premises, showing the size and present use of rooms
- sketch plans of the proposed work
- a specification of the work to be done

(If the cost is over a specified figure, this documentation must be prepared by an architect, surveyor or other qualified person.)

- *either* a statement from the local authority confirming that the project is not contrary to its development plans, building regulations or by-laws *or* copies of documents giving the relevant approvals
- if the property is leased, the landlord's written consent to alteration.

No application can be considered by the FHSA without this documentation.

How FHSAs deal with applications

If the FHSA decides that the GP's proposed alterations would significantly improve the existing premises, it will decide what priority to give the scheme within its overall programme for surgery improvements.

If a scheme is approved in principle the applicant will be told, and advised of the percentage reimbursement and of any conditions such as a target date or timeband for payment. The GP should confirm in writing whether he or she intends to go ahead with the scheme, and if proceeding should then obtain tenders. Three tenders are normally required and the grant is based on the lowest.

The FHSA will give approval for the work to start and ask the GP to complete an agreement form. *None of the grant can be paid until this agreement is completed.*

If a GP has to change the scheme in some way, the FHSA should be told immediately.

If a project is estimated to cost above a certain figure (*see* schedule 2 of the improvement grant section of the Red Book), instalments of the grant up to 90% of the estimated total may be paid if the GP asks for this arrangement when applying.

Before an instalment can be paid, the FHSA must see an architect's certificate showing project costs incurred so far. The instalment payment will be the approved proportion (between 33% to 66%) of the costs incurred.

When work is completed and the GP has made all payments, payment of the grant (or the remaining amount) should be claimed on a form supplied by the FHSA. When making the claim, the GP should also send receipted bills, details of the cost of any ineligible items and documents to substantiate any additional costs. The FHSA may wish an officer to visit and see the improvements before making the final payment.

Grants and tax allowances

The costs of work cannot qualify for both an improvement grant and a tax allowance; a practice should obtain its accountant's advice before deciding which would be more advantageous. If part of an improvement project does not qualify for a grant, the GP can seek tax relief on the residual costs.

Representations

If a practice disagrees with an FHSA's decision that a project is ineligible for a grant, it may appeal to the Secretary of State, explaining why it is dissatisfied.

Cost rent

A practice may opt for reimbursement related to the cost of providing separate purpose-built premises, or their equivalent, instead of a current market rent; this reimbursement is known as a 'cost rent'.

The FHSA considers applications in the context of its current policies and cash allocation; not all applications for cost rent schemes are approved, and for those that are, reimbursement may be conditional upon the project starting within a specific timescale.

Any of the following types of project may qualify for a cost rent:

- building completely new premises
- acquiring premises for substantial modification
- substantially modifying existing premises.

The premises may be owned or rented by the GP and the general provisions of the rent and rates scheme, including the requirement for acceptance by the FHSA and the possibility of abatement for private practice, apply.

The scheme gives financial assistance to doctors providing premises suitable for general medical services and appropriate supporting services.

When seeking reimbursement of a cost rent the GP must, before entering into any commitments, obtain FHSA approval of the project under the rent and rates scheme and an offer in writing:

- stating that the cost of the proposed project will be reimbursed on a cost rent basis
- specifying how the reimbursement will be calculated
- giving a preliminary estimate of the amount to be reimbursed (known as the interim cost rent)
- giving a target date when the reimbursement may start. (If a practice is unable to comply with an agreed timetable, the FHSA may withdraw approval; the practice would need to reapply for the scheme to continue and it would be responsible for any abortive expenses incurred.)

This written offer enables the practice to decide whether to proceed with the project or modify it; it should tell the FHSA whether it intends to proceed.

A practice should ensure that:

- it obtains good advice from the outset and the FHSA and its medical adviser are consulted about any proposal to build new or substantially improved premises
- an architect is appointed, preferably one familiar with designing surgery premises and the cost rent scheme (particularly its constraints on costs and room sizes)

- planning permission is obtained from the local authority before any substantial financial commitment is taken on
- it is aware when arranging finance that the prescribed percentage (*see* pages 136–137) to be applied to the accepted building cost, and the schedule costs applicable, will be those prevailing when a tender is accepted or a lease is signed
- where a doctor proposes leasing premises under a purchase and lease arrangement, agreement has been obtained from the lessor before any financial commitment is made
- it is aware reimbursement is paid only from the date when the premises are brought fully into use.

Some definitions

New separate purpose-built premises

These are newly-erected, designed according to the scheme's recommendations for overall size, size of individual rooms and costs, and used solely for practice purposes (apart from any residential accommodation for a message-taker).

Substantial alteration of premises

This should involve structural work such as extending or modifying a building, and:

- in the case of an extension, should provide additional accommodation at least equal to the area of a combined consulting and examination room and its associated circulation space, currently defined as 12.5 square metres;
- in the case of a modification without an extension, the structural work should cost at least the equivalent of the extension referred to above.

In both cases, the substantial alteration must in the FHSA's view make the surgery the equivalent of separate purpose-built premises.

Alterations will not qualify for a cost rent even if the cost exceeds the minimum cost specified, unless:

- the alteration involves the necessary structural work
- any additional accommodation is necessary.

Outline approval

This is approval in principle of the proposed scheme, stating what priority it will be given within the FHSA's overall programme and when reimbursement may be expected. It does not involve any firm financial commitment by the FHSA.

Written offer

This is the FHSA's formal offer of cost rent reimbursement and normally includes an estimate of the interim cost rent. An FHSA may however give a preliminary cost rent assessment, prior to a detailed interim calculation at a later date. *Doctors are advised not to enter into any financial commitment before receiving and accepting a written offer.*

Interim cost rent

This figure is calculated by the FHSA on the basis of the provisional site value, the cost schedules and the prescribed percentage. It enables the GP to decide whether the proposed project is financially sound before entering into any substantial commitments.

Actual cost of site

This is the amount paid for the site, including VAT.

Prescribed percentage

This is the rate of reimbursement used to compute the final cost rent payable. It is determined as follows:

- For owner-occupiers, the prescribed percentage is the rate of interest on the date the GP accepts the tender for the project. The appropriate rate will be the variable reimbursement rate notified by the Department except that:
  - ▽ if the GP is financing a scheme wholly or mainly on a fixed rate basis, the prescribed percentage will be the fixed reimbursement rate
  - ▽ if the GP is financing a scheme wholly or mainly through a fixed loan but with the option to switch to a variable interest rate loan, the prescribed percentage will be the fixed rate unless and until the GP opts to switch to a variable rate, in which case the prescribed percentage will be the variable rate from the date when it takes effect
  - ▽ if the GP is financing the scheme wholly or mainly from his or her own funds, the prescribed percentage will be the fixed reimbursement rate.
- If the prescribed percentage is the variable reimbursement rate, the final cost rent will be altered subsequently in line with changes in the rate.
- If a GP leases premises from a third party, the prescribed percentage will be the fixed reimbursement rate prevailing when the main lease is signed. If leased premises are subsequently extended, the prescribed percentage on the extension will be the rate prevailing when the lease on the extension (or the amended lease on the extended property) is signed.

So that the FHSA can work out the appropriate rate of interest in order to calculate the cost rent, a GP should tell it how the scheme is to be financed before tenders are signed. If the financing arrangements are not settled at that time the FHSA should be told as soon as they are known – certainly no later than six months after signing the contract.

Final cost rent

This is based on the costs of the project finally approved by the FHSA; these will be the costs incurred, providing these are allowable under the scheme and do not exceed its total cost limits. The actual cost rent will be calculated by applying the prescribed percentage to the approved cost.

If the appropriate prescribed percentage is the variable reimbursement rate, the FHSA will alter the cost rent payable whenever the variable rate changes.

Schedule cost (unit cost limit)

The schedules in the Red Book indicate the upper limits (excluding site costs) of payment for new separate purpose built premises; they are intended to make reasonable provision for a good standard of accommodation. The schedules are reviewed annually and amended to reflect changes in building costs. For owner-occupied premises, the date on which schedule costs are calculated is the date the tender is accepted, and for leased premises the date the main lease is signed.

Actual rent

This is the rent actually paid by a GP to a landlord.

Operative date for reimbursement

This is the first day on which the new or modified surgery is brought fully into use.

Current market value of site

This is the value of the site on the open market, assuming that it is available for development for any purpose for which planning permission might reasonably be expected.

Third parties

For the purpose of the scheme third parties exclude:

- members of a GP's family
- private companies of which he or she, or any partner, or a member of his or her or their families is a shareholder. (An application involving such a company will only qualify for exemption if the doctor or partner or family member individually or collectively holds a majority of the shares)
- charitable trusts established for the relief of sickness or the preservation or protection of health, of which part of the trust's activities may be to make premises available to GPs at a full commercial rate for use as a surgery.

Similar conditions apply to all these exclusions as to doctors who are owner-occupiers.

General guidance

Siting of premises and standards

Advice on standards of accommodation is given in paragraph 56 schedule 1 of the Red Book. When choosing a site for new premises, a GP should bear in mind the possibility that extra expense may be incurred because of site conditions. For instance the site may be uneven, marshy, or have suspect subsoil strata.

When a site is chosen, the GP should seek outline approval for the proposed project from the FHSA. It will assess the proposal against its priorities for premises and decide whether it is acceptable under the rent and rates scheme. The FHSA will also provide an estimate of when cost rent payments can be expected.

The FHSA will consider an additional allowance if a site involving exceptional expenditure on site work has had to be chosen.

Before buying a site a GP must ensure that the local authority will grant planning permission (or at least outline permission) for practice premises to be built.

The FHSA should be given as much information as possible about the site, including its price, a plan of its layout, and the tenure arrangements (whether freehold or leasehold, and if leasehold, the ground rent and length of lease). The FHSA and district valuer will need to know of any restrictive covenants, easements, rights of way, fixed charges, or special outgoings other than normal rates or taxes. The district valuer's valuation depends on all this information about the site.

If a site larger than that required for the practice is purchased, reimbursement will be based on the total site cost (or the district valuer's valuation, whichever is lower) but the FHSA will encourage the practice to dispose of any excess land.

Architect's sketch plans

These should show the dimensions of the premises, and the size and proposed use of each room. They should be sent to the FHSA.

Self supply and VAT registration

After 1 August 1989, any doctor developing new premises where the project has a total cost (including land) of more than £100 000 must register for VAT. Self supply occurs when a doctor supplies premises to himself or herself on completion of the project or on first occupation, whichever is sooner. The doctor is classed as a developer of new premises, and the self supply is subject to VAT at the standard rate.

A doctor or partnership must apply to the local VAT office for registration within 30 days of the self supply, otherwise a financial penalty may be imposed. If registration is undertaken at the start of the development, cash flow can be improved by recovering VAT paid out to contractors and professional advisers.

Advice should be obtained from an accountant on the registration procedure and completion of quarterly VAT returns (which must be submitted promptly to avoid penalties for late submission). VAT paid out on the project during development (including any incurred on services received during the six months prior to registration) can be recovered. This includes VAT paid on the land cost as well as on goods and services, but not any VAT paid in connection with the provision of health care.

At the time of the self supply, VAT must be paid on the total value of the project. When all the VAT paid out on the project has been reclaimed, the doctor or partnership should then deregister. In the final analysis, VAT will have been levied on all the costs of the project at the standard rate.

The FHSA's role

Site

The district valuer will give the FHSA an assessment of the site's current market value.

The cost schedules

The cost schedules (paragraph 51 schedule 1 of the Red Book) specify the upper limits on what the FHSA will pay for new separate purpose-built premises (or their equivalent). The limits include VAT but not site cost. The schedules are intended to enable a good standard surgery premises to be built. They take account of the number of doctors likely to be consulting at the same time. The number of consulting rooms need not equal the number of doctors in the practice.

If a trainee practitioner is regularly employed, an additional suite may be provided, but will not be accepted as part of the practice unit. The formula applying to an optional additional room will be used to calculate the cost rent. The FHSA may also approve additional rooms for attached staff such as district nurses and health visitors.

Variations from recommended sizes

Doctors may build premises larger than those permitted according to the schedules, but the building cost limits will not be increased. FHSAs may also agree to areas smaller than those specified in the schedules provided the individual rooms conform to the minimum size standards.

However, if existing buildings are being modified, the FHSA will exercise discretion in applying cost limit reductions if the room sizes and the overall building size differ from the schedule figures because of the dimensions of the original building.

Calculating the cost limits

FHSAs calculate the notional cost of the building work by comparing the area of the proposed surgery premises with that specified in the schedule. Minor differences may be ignored, but the cost limits for the practice will be increased to take account of training facilities and reduced if the area proposed is at least 5% less than the area in the appropriate schedule. (Paragraph 51.52.13 of the Red Book explains how this is done.)

To the cost of the practice unit, FHSAs add the cost of any optional additional rooms, and to the aggregate of both a percentage is added to cover external works, the preparation of car parks etc., site work and off-site work. To the aggregate of all these figures is added a further percentage for professional fees. The cost limit is subject to the regional variations shown in paragraph 51 schedule 1 of the Red Book; each FHSA area is allocated to one of four bands which reflect variations in building costs, as shown in paragraph 51 schedule 3.

Message-taker's accommodation

If a GP wishes to include in a cost rent scheme residential accommodation occupied by someone (other than a doctor) who takes calls from patients outside surgery hours, the FHSA should be consulted before any plans are drawn up. The FHSA may approve such accommodation if it considers it reasonable to do so, and the costs allowed will be those of an optional additional room.

Interim cost rent

The FHSA will advise the GP of the interim cost rent, which is the prescribed percentage of:

- the site value (or the market value of the site only if premises are to be bought for modification) as assessed by the district valuer, or the actual site cost, whichever is lower; and
- the schedule cost (or the equivalent) of the proposed project.

The interim cost rent is based on figures prevailing at the time it is calculated; subsequent changes in the prescribed percentage and the schedule cost will be taken account of in the final cost rent.

Subsequent variations

The FHSA must be told as soon as possible of any significant changes to the information originally provided – for example the sale of part of the site or a change in the plans – so that it can approve the changes and if necessary recalculate the interim cost rent.

Tenders

FHSAs normally expect GPs to provide three tenders for building work. However, if this causes significant difficulties, two may be accepted, or even one if the FHSA gives its prior agreement.

GPs should seek tenders on a firm price basis and confirm that quoted items such as prime cost sums are realistic and reasonable provision has been made for contingencies. Firm price tenders, however, do allow increases in costs due to government policy – for example, changes in taxation.

If exceptionally a GP cannot obtain a fixed price tender because the project is expected to take more than a year to complete, the FHSA will consider accepting a price fluctuation clause for cost rent purposes providing it approves this before the building contract is signed.

Current market rent

The cost rent for new or substantially modified premises is an alternative to current market rent. Initially, it is unlikely that current market rent will yield more reimbursement than a cost rent. Unless a GP believes current market rent could exceed cost rent, he or she should not ask for an assessment of current market rent when a new scheme commences. The cost rent will be paid until the GP chooses to change, on a review, to current market rent, or until the premises or a significant part of them cease to be used for practice purposes.

Reviews can be carried out:

- for premises owned by GPs, every three years from the operative date of the cost rent; and
- for premises leased by GPs, when a review of the rent is due under the terms of the lease, or a new lease is entered into at the end of the existing lease.

Improvement grants

An improvement grant may be claimed when substantially improving premises through the cost rent scheme. Any grant paid will be deducted from the aggregate cost to which the prescribed percentage is applied.

Unusual projects

Proposed projects which the FHSA accepts as designed to produce the equivalent of separate purpose-built premises but which are not specifically covered by the cost rent scheme, have to be referred to the Department of Health for advice on how to calculate a cost rent.

Specific procedures

Paragraphs 51.53.1 to 51.58.21 of the Red Book explain how FHSAs calculate the final cost rent in various circumstances. Two typical examples show how this is done.

Example 1: new premises to be owned by the practice

The final cost rent will be the prescribed percentage of the aggregate of:

- the actual cost of the site when acquired by the GP or its current market value at the date of assessment by the district valuer, whichever is less
- fees and legal costs arising from the purchase of the site, including the legal costs of obtaining a mortgage
- the cost (based on the lowest acceptable tender) of building work (including professional fees) or the notional cost for this work based on the appropriate cost limits, whichever is less
- where, before completion of premises, loans are obtained to buy the site or to finance progress payments (to the value of the work done as certified by an architect), interest charged on these loans up to the operative date of the cost rent reimbursement.

Example 2: substantial modification of existing premises owned by the practice

The final cost rent will be:

either a combination of the reassessed current market rent or the existing rent of the original premises, whichever is larger, and a cost rent calculated as the prescribed percentage of the aggregate of:

- the cost of adaptation (including actual professional fees) and the cost of any additional land or premises acquired by the doctor *or* their value as assessed by the district valuer, whichever is less
- the statutory cost of passing plans and first inspection of the building
- fees and legal costs arising from purchase of the additional land and premises including, where applicable, the legal costs of obtaining a mortgage, and
- where, before completion of the adaptation, loans are obtained to buy additional land or premises or finance progress payments (to the value of work done as certified by an architect), interest charged on these loans to the operative date of the final cost rent reimbursement

or the prescribed percentage of the aggregate of:

- the value of the site and premises at the date of acquisition by the GP as assessed by the district valuer *plus* whichever is the less of the value of any additional land and premises similarly assessed *or* their actual cost
- the appropriate unit cost for new purpose-built premises of the same size as the existing premises after adaptation
- fees and legal costs arising from the purchase of the additional land and premises including, where applicable, the legal costs of obtaining a mortgage, and
- where, before completion of the adaptation, loans are obtained to buy additional land or finance progress payments (to the value of work done as certified by an architect), interest charged on these loans to the operative date of the final cost rent reimbursement,

whichever is less.

Ground rent

The FHSA should be told if a site is leasehold when the GP is applying for approval. When the work has been completed a copy of the lease showing the ground rent payable should be sent to the FHSA, together with the other documents required at that stage.

The ground rent will be included in the final cost rent calculations unless it has already been included in a current market rent assessment.

Purchase and lease

Under a purchase and lease scheme, a bank, building society or other reputable financial institution may acquire from a practice newly-completed, self-contained, purpose-built surgery accommodation or its equivalent if this does not include residential accommodation for the doctors and is separately assessed for rating. The financial institution may then lease these premises back to the doctors. Paragraph 51.58 of the Red Book describes this scheme.

31 Health centres

SPECIAL financial arrangements apply to GPs in health centres. A health centre is defined as premises owned by the Department of Health and managed by a health authority, within which accommodation is provided for GPs. DHAs are responsible for health centres, and in consultation with FHSAs will make financial arrangements for their use by GPs.

Charges to GPs

Charges cover:

- rent of accommodation
- a contribution in lieu of rates and water rates or water meter charges
- practice staff employed by the health authority who work for the GPs
- services such as heating, hot water, lighting, cleaning, internal repairs and decorations, furniture, moveable equipment and telephones (including the cost of staff providing these services).

Because the first three categories of charges are usually reimbursed directly, they are treated separately from those under the fourth category.

Box 31.1: Health centre charges

- charges for rent and rates are fully reimbursed
- charges for any practice staff provided by the health authority may be partially or wholly reimbursed by the FHSA, according to the practice staff scheme
- charges for services such as heating, lighting and cleaning are not directly reimbursed

---

Accounting

Most GPs in health centres have their rent and rates, together with the costs of any health authority employed staff, reimbursed at the same time as expenditure is incurred.

Although these costs are directly reimbursed, they still count as outgoings and should be recorded as such in GPs' tax returns, which are available for the Inland Revenue survey of expenses which provides key evidence to the Doctors' and Dentists' Review Body. The FHSA should advise GPs working in health centres at least annually of any notional charges paid directly on their behalf. GPs must ensure that the first amount is shown gross as expenditure in their accounts and the second as income in the same way as capitation fees and other receipts.

Arrangements for payment

The arrangements for paying health centre costs and charges vary. Some practices pay the whole of these charges directly to the health authority and subsequently claim reimbursement from the FHSA, while others have these charges (less any reimbursable amounts) deducted from their remuneration by the FHSA, so that they can be paid directly to the DHA.

Accommodation charges

In order to agree appropriate charges for accommodation, the FHSA confirms with the health authority and GPs the amount of accommodation used exclusively or primarily by the GPs, and the amount used jointly with other health centre users – for example a waiting room. This information may also affect service charges.

Contribution in lieu of rates

The same information about room usage is used by the FHSA and DHA to calculate the contribution due in lieu of rates, which is also reimbursable.

Assessing the rent

The district valuer assesses the current market rent of the practice's share of the accommodation using the agreed information on usage. The only exception applies to those health centres in use before 1 April 1974 for which a cost rent was calculated. Accommodation charges are normally reviewed every three years.

Practice staff

Most GPs in health centres employ their own staff and are reimbursed in the normal way. A health authority should not charge GPs for attached professional staff, such as district nurses, midwives and health visitors.

If a health authority provides GPs with clerical or administrative staff it should agree with the GPs both the details of the duties to be undertaken and the charges to be made. The practice can claim reimbursement of these charges under the practice staff scheme.

Private work in health centres

GPs doing private work in health centres must obtain permission from the FHSA. It will want to know how much private income is being earned, in order to determine whether the amounts reimbursed for accommodation, rates and staff should be abated.

Service charges

These charges should be agreed between the practice and DHA, in consultation with the FHSA. The charges for services and for practice staff will be adjusted if the full cost is more than that which would be incurred by a practice for similar facilities in privately owned premises in the locality.

Box 31.2: Service charges

Service charges can be compared with those incurred by GPs practising outside health centres in comparable premises

---

Arbitration

Any dispute about health centre charges may be settled by arbitration as provided for in a health centre licence. Even if no licence has been agreed, a health authority will probably agree to the type of arbitration referred to in the Model Health Centre Licence issued in 1977 by the Department of Health and Social Security.

32 Practice staff

THE practice staff scheme introduced on 1 April 1990 replaced the former ancillary staff scheme; it significantly changed the arrangements for reimbursing GPs' practice staff costs.

Many of the rules of the previous scheme, which virtually guaranteed reimbursement, have been abolished; FHSAs now have greater discretion, particularly in relation to categories of staff which can be included and how much should be reimbursed.

Under the practice staff scheme, there is no longer a restrictive definition of 'qualifying staff' and a GP can therefore claim payment for a wider range of staff, including physiotherapists, chiropodists, dietitians, counsellors, linkworkers and translators. There is also no limit on the total number of staff for which a GP can claim reimbursement and no bar on reimbursing the costs of employing relatives and dependents.

The FHSA is required to publish a policy on the use of its cash limited resources for practice staff, which informs GPs of priorities and the likelihood of a particular post attracting reimbursement. The health needs of patients must be a key factor in determining how an FHSA targets its resources.

General outline

The scheme provides for direct reimbursement at FHSA discretion of all or part of the expense of employing practice staff (excluding those employed to undertake medical duties such as GP trainees and assistants). Any remaining balance of expenditure on staff is reimbursed indirectly to the profession as a whole through the expenses element of gross fees and allowances.

The FHSA exercises its discretion according to the constraints outlined below; it has to work within an overall cash limit set annually by the Department of Health. Some parts will therefore attract no reimbursement at all.

All GPs, including those providing restricted services or with limited lists, are eligible for reimbursement, subject to FHSA discretion.

Payment

The GP may be reimbursed directly any proportion of any one or more of the following staff costs:

- practice staff salaries

- gross national insurance contributions paid by the employer (i.e. the total sum due before deducting any employer's NI refund for statutory sick pay (SSP) and statutory maternity pay (SMP))
- contributions paid by the employer to the NHS superannuation scheme or an approved private superannuation scheme
- cost of providing practice staff training (including course fees and travel and subsistence expenses)
- payments to an agency, including a health authority, excluding the agency's administrative or overhead costs
- the balance between the total payment due under the Employment Protection (Consolidation) Act 1978 and any rebate paid by the Department of Employment, where a GP is required by the Act to make a redundancy payment to an employee whose salary costs have been previously reimbursed (an FHSA will withhold payment towards these costs if a GP acted without due regard to the FHSA's responsibilities)
- payment of salary for reasonable amounts of paid holiday, sick leave, maternity leave and training, excluding any payments made under the SSP or SMP schemes
- payment of salary for relief staff (which may include practice staff covering for absent colleagues) employed to cover staff during holidays, sick leave, maternity leave and training.

Definitions

Salary: the gross amount of basic pay before deducting income tax, national insurance, any superannuation or private pension scheme contribution, but excluding any SSP or SMP payments. It does not include overtime payments or emoluments in kind, but can include payments for providing cover for other staff.

Post: an appointment which, once approved by the FHSA, normally continues to be reimbursed at a similar level unless there is a significant change in local circumstances on review. GPs may, however, also seek approval for short term or temporary posts.

Post-holder: a person appointed to fill a specific post.

Staff training

Claims for reimbursement of training costs must have prior approval. Costs may include approved proportions of course fees and travel and subsistence expenses. The FHSA will not reimburse the training costs of agency staff (except for health authority administrative staff working for GPs in a health centre), or of attached health authority staff such as district nurses or health visitors.

How to apply for direct reimbursement

Practices may apply for reimbursement for either directly employed staff or certain agency staff. The FHSA may approve applications, in whole or part, or may refuse them entirely. The FHSA has discretion to decide:

- the percentage of salary, salary increase, or any other payment which should be directly reimbursed
- the date from which reimbursement will be made
- the minimum qualifications and experience required of practice staff
- the percentage of practice staff training costs to be reimbursed
- how to review its reimbursement of posts, no more often than every three years.

Key features of a practice's application and the FHSA's periodic reviews are:

- a job description setting out responsibilities, roles and objectives
- an employment contract including salary review arrangements (e.g. annual increments and cost of living increases).

When deciding on the percentage of costs to be directly reimbursed, an FHSA must take account of its plans for developing GP services, its cash limit, the circumstances of individual practices – for example any local recruitment or retention problems – and the need to deal fairly and consistently with practices in similar circumstances over the years.

The FHSA should explain to the practice how it intends to review the post periodically.

Applications, notifications and claims should be submitted on the forms listed in Box 32.1.

Arrangements for staff in post on 31 March 1990 to whom special transitional arrangements still apply are described below. In all other circumstances, a practice planning to increase the amount to be reimbursed or the salary level (even if there is no overall increase in reimbursement because the cost is off-set by reducing the hours worked) should seek prior approval using form FP/PS1, unless the FHSA has relaxed this requirement and asked for notification on form FP/PS3. This relaxation could apply where the FHSA notifies practices of the maximum amount it regards as a reasonable cost of living increase: lesser increases would then not require prior approval, and a practice only needs to submit form FP/PS1 if it wishes to be reimbursed for an increase above that already approved by the FHSA.

Practices should normally apply on form FP/PS1 for direct reimbursement for a particular post in which specified duties are undertaken, rather than for a specified post-holder. If the post-holder subsequently changes there is no need to submit a further application unless the practice seeks increased reimbursement to reflect enhanced duties, a change of hours or salary, or to fill a post which has been vacant for more than three months.

Box 32.1: Practice staff scheme forms

- application for prior approval for all new posts   FP/PS1
- application for any increase in the cost of existing staff to be directly reimbursed
- application for any significant change in the hours or nature of duties of existing staff

- application for prior approval for reimbursement of   FP/PS2
  expenses for attendance at training events

- notification of change of post-holder (including details of   FP/PS3
  new post-holder) and dates of commencement and
  termination of employment
- notification of change of salary level (in circumstances
  described in paragraph 52.13)
- notification of any reduction in the cost to be directly
  reimbursed, for example reduction in salary levels or hours

- claims for reimbursement (including claims for attendance   FP/PS4
  at training events)

Applications for prior approval on form FP/PS1 should be submitted no later than six weeks before the intended date of employment, or by any other date decided by the FHSA. Applications for approval for direct reimbursement of expenses for practice staff training should be submitted on form FP/PS2 as far in advance as possible.

Notifying the start or end of employment

A change of post-holder, or the commencement or termination of employment of practice staff, should be notified to the FHSA on form FP/PS3 as soon as possible, and no later than 14 days after the change.

Submitting claims and receiving payments

Claims for reimbursement should be submitted quarterly on form FP/PS4, within 10 days of the end of the quarter. Payments are normally made quarterly. In the case of directly employed staff, form FP/PS4 should be signed by them; for agency staff a receipt from the agency should be submitted.

Payments will be abated if more than 10% of a GP's income comes from private practice.

The FHSA may make monthly payments in advance.

Practice accounts

GPs should record total staff expenses as gross expenditure and direct reimbursements as income in their accounts, so that reliable data are available in the Inland Revenue's annual survey of practice expenses for the Review Body.

Staff qualifications

The minimum qualifications and experience which FHSAs regard as necessary for practice staff reflect the standards adopted by either national professional regulatory bodies or organizations awarding recognized vocational qualifications. In the case of administrative and clerical staff, the FHSA may use its discretion and must take account of qualifications or experience normally expected of these staff for whom in-service training may be appropriate. The FHSA may also specify a reasonable time span within which a new member of staff should be able to acquire a core level of competence necessary for the job.

Paragraph 52.23 of the Red Book describes the qualifications of a practice nurse (normally a registered general nurse) and the extra qualifications required for nurses undertaking special duties such as midwifery, health visiting and district nursing. A practice nurse who is an enrolled nurse may undertake only a limited range of duties.

The periodic review

All posts approved after 31 March 1990, and previous posts to which the transitional arrangements have ceased to apply, are reviewed no more often than every three years. Although an FHSA may stop reimbursement following a review, it must act consistently and reasonably, taking account of the continuing need for experienced and skilled practice staff.

Transitional arrangements

Those staff employed prior to 1 April 1990 under the former ancillary staff scheme are exempted from the new practice staff scheme unless a practice:

- applies to increase the amount directly reimbursed: e.g. to reflect increased working hours, an increased proportion of salary or other costs directly reimbursed or an increased salary (apart from a reasonable salary increase which the FHSA has approved, or any reasonable annual scale increment to which the employee has been contractually entitled prior to

1 April 1990 or an increase in employer's national insurance contributions, or contributions paid by the employer to the NHS superannuation scheme or a qualifying superannuation scheme)
- applies to modify substantially the duties of the post
- applies for reimbursement of the employee's training expenses.

Applications relating to the first two situations above should be made on form FP/PS1, and to the third on form FP/PS2. In all cases, claims for direct reimbursement should be submitted on form FP/PS4.

Practice staff in post on 31 March 1990 for whom the FHSA had already agreed to make reimbursements, are not subject to periodic reviews unless their hours or duties change substantially or they leave. From then on, the direct reimbursement arrangements applying to the subsequent post-holder are subject to review. Since the FHSA normally reviews immediately whether there is a case for continued reimbursement, a practice should consult the FHSA before recruiting a successor.

Practice staff employed by health authorities in health centres

The arrangements for practice staff employed by health authorities in health centres are explained on page 146.

A proportion of computer costs, incurred by a principal, restricted principal, partnership or group practice, can be directly reimbursed under a cash-limited scheme started on 1 April 1990. The costs of purchasing, leasing, upgrading and maintaining a computer system, and the initial staff costs of setting it up, are all eligible for direct reimbursement. Any remaining expenditure is reimbursed indirectly. Claims which are not reimbursed because funds are not available may be resubmitted the following year.

Definitions

Hardware includes computers and associated equipment, but excludes any computer which is an integral part of another piece of equipment, single-function word processors and telephone lines, except dedicated lines linking computers in main and branch surgeries.

Software refers to computer programs principally used for practice administration and patient care.

Upgrading refers to enhancing an existing system's functions to improve patient care or administrative efficiency.

Which expenses are covered by the scheme?

Purchase costs

If a practice pays the full cost of purchasing and installing a system, hardware and software costs can be directly reimbursed, less any deduction for private income from the sale of anonymized data. Normally up to 50% of the cost is reimbursed, except for fund-holders, to whom 75% of hardware costs and 100% of software and training costs may be reimbursed. If a practice chooses to purchase a system it previously leased, the total reimbursement of leasing and purchase costs is normally limited to the same percentages of the original cost of the system.

Leasing costs

Leasing costs can be directly reimbursed, less any deduction for private income from the sale of anonymized data. Normally up to 50% of the cost is reimbursed, except for fund-holders, who may receive reimbursement of 75% of hardware costs and 100% of software costs. However, doctors who were already receiving leasing payments for computers obtained before 22 July 1991 continue to receive at least the level of reimbursement they were getting on 21 July 1991, which was subject to a sliding scale related to list size.

Upgrading costs

If the practice pays the full cost of an upgrade, either by purchasing or leasing, a proportion of the hardware and software costs may be reimbursed, less any deduction for private income from the sale of anonymized data, and irrespective of whether the existing system is owned, rented or leased. The normal limits on direct reimbursement are as described above under the headings purchase costs and leasing costs.

Maintenance costs

A proportion of the costs of maintaining the hardware and software of a computer system, less any deduction for private income from the sale of anonymized data, can be reimbursed irrespective of when the system was purchased. If maintenance is included in a leasing agreement but not separately identified, and is already being reimbursed via the reimbursement of leasing costs, no additional payment is due. Normally up to 50% of the costs are reimbursed, except for fund-holders, who may receive reimbursement of 75% of hardware costs and 100% of software costs. However, doctors who were already receiving maintenance payments for computers obtained before 22 July 1991 continue to receive at least the level of reimbursement they were getting on 21 July 1991, which was subject to a sliding scale related to list size.

Staff costs

Up to 70% of the staff costs incurred in setting up a computer system may be directly reimbursed. These costs cannot also be claimed under the practice staff scheme.

How to claim

Claims for system purchase costs should be submitted on form CM1; those for leasing costs on form CM2, either annually or monthly depending on how often costs are incurred; claims for upgrading are sent on form CM3; those for maintenance costs on form CM4, either annually or monthly depending on when payments are made; and claims for staff costs are submitted on form CM5. The following documents should be sent with each claim: receipts for purchases and upgrades; copies of agreements for leasing and maintenance claims; and a contract of employment, stating the job description, period of employment and salary paid, with staff cost claims (*see* Box 33.1). Details of any private income from the sale of anonymized data should also be sent with forms CM1, 2, 3 and 4.

Box 33.1: Computer cost claims		
costs claimed	form	additional documents required
purchase costs	CM1	receipt
leasing costs	CM2	leasing agreement
upgrading costs	CM3	receipt
maintenance costs	CM4	maintenance agreement
initial staff costs	CM5	employment contract

Because the scheme is cash limited, FHSAs have discretion to take account of the effects of computerization on patient care and administrative efficiency and the need to apply consistent criteria to different practices. Practices should consult FHSAs before submitting claims.

Appeals

A GP who disagrees with an FHSA's decision may appeal to the Secretary of State within two months.

34 Payment arrangements

THE 'responsible' FHSA normally makes all payments to which a GP is entitled apart from rural practice payments, which may be made by the FHSA that determines eligibility for these payments even though it is not the GP's 'responsible' FHSA. The 'responsible' FHSA will obtain from any other FHSAs in whose lists a GP or his or her partners are also included the information needed to determine eligibility to receive:

- basic practice allowance and related allowances
- allowances for employing associate doctors and locums employed by rural single-handed GPs on study leave
- payments during sickness, confinement and prolonged study leave
- capitation fees, deprivation payments and child health surveillance fees
- inducement payments and initial practice allowances
- rural practice payments (except as described above)
- registration fees and payments for minor surgery sessions, health promotion and chronic disease management
- target payments for vaccinations and immunizations and cervical cytology
- students allowance
- payments under trainee practitioner scheme
- doctor's retainer scheme sessional payments
- postgraduate education allowance
- reimbursement for staff and premises
- reimbursement of computer costs.

GPs should claim the following fees from the FHSA for the locality where a patient lives or is temporarily residing, or in the case of emergency treatment for the locality where it is provided:

- maternity medical services fees
- contraceptive services fees
- night visit fees
- temporary resident fees
- emergency treatment fees
- immediately necessary treatment fees
- fees for the arrest of dental haemorrhage
- anaesthetists' fees
- vaccination and immunization fees.

The FHSAs receiving claims check them and notify the responsible FHSA of the amounts to be paid.

Box 34.1: Payment arrangements

All fees and allowances are paid by the responsible FHSA except, in some circumstances, rural practice payments. However, some claims have to be submitted to the FHSA for the area where a patient lives

---

Capitation fees, deprivation payments, child health surveillance fees and practice allowances will be paid no later than the last day of the quarter in which they are due.

Claims for most item of service fees (night visits, vaccinations etc.) are accepted if made within six months of the service being provided, or in the case of MMS within six months of the expected date of confinement if this is later. Practices should submit claims as quickly as possible.

The FHSA may accept claims made up to six years after the service was provided; its decision will depend on why the delay occurred. Only the Secretary of State can exceptionally approve claims after six years.

Box 34.2: Submitting claims

- item-of-service claims must be submitted within six months of when the service was provided
- FHSAs have discretion to accept claims made within six years

---

Arrangements for making provisional payments or withholding payments where eligibility is in doubt are described in paragraph 75.6. The arrangements for paying dispensing doctors are in paragraph 75.7.

If two or more practitioners are in partnership:

- claims for services provided by either or any of them may be submitted as a single claim in the name of the partnership
- payments may, if the partners wish, be made as a single payment to the partnership.

Advances on account

Advance payment can be obtained for capitation fees, child health surveillance, deprivation payments, allowances and certain payments under the trainee practitioner scheme. Advances may be made either:

- midway in the quarter, when the advance will not exceed half the estimated payments for the quarter, or
- monthly, when the advance will not exceed one-third of the estimated payments for the quarter.

Advances can also be claimed for rural practice payments, temporary resident fees, rent and rates and practice staff payments. Advance payments improve a practice's cash flow; GPs should ensure they claim these and review them regularly so as to reflect increases in practice income.

Box 34.3: Advances on account

- advances can be made for most FHSA payments, including direct reimbursements
- advances improve a practice's cash flow

---

35 Appeals to the Secretary of State

GPs who disagree with an FHSA decision may appeal to the Secretary of State. (The actual term used in the Red Book is 'making representations'.)

A separate appeal system exists for the rent and rates scheme. For all other appeals, a GP who is dissatisfied with a decision on remuneration must send relevant information to the FHSA. If the FHSA does not alter its decision the GP may then appeal to the Secretary of State. This must be done as soon as possible after receiving the FHSA's final decision. The GP must submit a case to the Secretary of State explaining the grounds of the appeal.

If a doctor is dissatisfied with an FHSA decision about an application or claim which has been refused on the grounds of the FHSA's management of its cash allocation, or about a health promotion or chronic disease management programme, representations can only be made on the grounds that the FHSA failed to follow Red Book procedures or failed to take account of material written evidence.

36 How the Red Book is negotiated and implemented

THE General Medical Services Committee (GMSC), a standing committee of the BMA with full authority to deal with all matters affecting NHS GPs, is the only body that represents all GPs irrespective of whether they are BMA members (although around 75% are). It is recognized as the GPs' sole negotiating body by the Department of Health. The GMSC is ultimately responsible for determining the advice to be given and representations to be made to ministers and government officials. Although the GMSC has final responsibility for determining the policies to be followed in negotiations, these cannot be formulated in a vacuum. It therefore convenes annually (and on other special occasions) a conference of LMC representatives. Over 300 GPs attend these conferences; they are not confined to BMA members because LMCs represent all GPs locally, just as the GMSC does at national level. The resolutions of these conferences are referred to the GMSC and provide the basis of its policy. It is said that the GMSC ignores conference policy at its peril.

In negotiations with ministers and government officials, the GMSC is represented by a negotiating team of five of its members, who are all working GPs. These doctors provide a direct input of their everyday experience of general practice into national negotiations, and are assisted by expert economic, industrial relations, legal and accountancy advisers. There is a regular cycle of meetings between the GMSC negotiating team and a team of Health Department officials, and these are supplemented by many other meetings to deal with specific matters. The experience of the GMSC's negotiating team has provided the Department of Health with invaluable advice on the practical implementations of its plans for the family doctor service, and LMCs have provided FHSAs with equally valuable advice.

Over the years negotiations between the GMSC and the Department of Health have covered a wide range of issues. In practice, the satisfactory completion of negotiations has only occasionally resulted in major amendments of the Red Book, while amendment of the legal framework of general practice, the NHS Regulations (which include the GP's terms of service), is rarer still. It is important to note that the Red Book, although a part of the NHS Regulations, can be amended without legislation, whereas the NHS Regulations are parliamentary enactments and thus require legislation to amend their provisions.

Consultation with the LMC: the traditional pattern

Because NHS GPs are independent contractors and not employees, successive governments recognized that special arrangements were required for administering the contracts GPs held with FPCs, the forerunners of today's FHSAs. Thus, the LMC nominated GPs for appointment by the Secretary of State for Health to serve with lay people and members of the other contractor professions as members of the FPC. The FPC members who were also working GPs brought a particular experience and expertise to the FPC. Through this representation, the day-to-day work of the FPC in its dealings with GPs was firmly based on the partnership principle. The term 'partnership principle' referred to an underlying presumption that LMCs and FPCs co-operated as equals to ensure GP services were run efficiently. Consensus and co-operation normally underlay the decisions reached and the manner in which they were implemented. The professional representation on the FPC itself was distinct from, and no substitute for, the process of consultation between FPCs and LMCs.

FPCs were required by statute to consult LMCs on many issues; this is still evident today in relation to FHSAs, in the Regulations governing the provision of NHS general medical services, the terms of service of GPs and the Statement of Fees and Allowances (the Red Book) (*see* Boxes 36.1 to 36.3). The LMC also continues to play an important part in the 'complaints procedure' and in the investigation of matters relating to professional conduct.

Box 36.1: Examples of references in the Regulations to consultation with the LMC

The LMC is to be consulted:

- before removal from the medical list of the name of a doctor who has personally never provided services or has ceased to provide services for the past six months
- on temporary arrangements for carrying on a practice
- where it appears that a doctor is incapable of providing general medical services because of his or her physical or mental condition
- on the termination of a maternity medical services contract where the doctor and the patient do not agree

---

Box 36.2: Examples of references in the terms of service to consultation with the LMC

The LMC is to be consulted:

- before the FHSA refuses consent or imposes conditions on a doctor's use of a deputizing service
- before refusing or withdrawing consent to employ an assistant
- in the inspection of surgery premises

Box 36.3: Examples of references in the Red Book to consultation with the LMC

- payment of a higher night visit fee
- acceptance of premises for rent and rates reimbursement
- the payment of delayed or late claims

The above examples are only illustrative. The extent of past LMC involvement in the day-to-day running of NHS general practice through its participation in the work of the FPC has been evident from the fact that the LMC was specifically referred to in over 20 paragraphs of the Regulations, 10 paragraphs of the terms of service and in over 30 paragraphs of the Red Book.

On many matters on which the FPC consulted the LMC, the two bodies jointly determined what action should be taken and in this sense 'consultation' meant 'partnership'. The local recognition and representation ensured the efficient provision of general medical services, enabling FPCs to draw upon the goodwill and experience of local GPs. The process of consultation also ensured that the terms of service negotiated centrally by the GMSC and Department of Health were fairly and reasonably applied locally, and that local discretion was properly exercised when implementing nationally agreed terms of service.

This relationship has now undergone radical change as described below.

The imposition of the 1990 contract

The imposition of new contractual arrangements, together with other managerial changes emanating from the Government's White Paper *Working for Patients*, created a very different climate of relations between the GMSC and the Department of Health, and between LMCs and FHSAs.

At national level, after many months of consultation, involving a measure of negotiation, the Government imposed new contractual arrangements on an unwilling and hostile profession. In doing so it consciously broke with a long tradition (extending back to the beginnings of the family doctor service in 1913) of proceeding by consensus, introducing contractual changes only after agreement with representatives of the profession.

However, during the past three years, relations at national level between the professions's representatives and ministers and their officials have steadily returned to normality and successful negotiations have been achieved in several areas.

At local level, relations between LMCs and FHSAs are undergoing a permanent and far more fundamental change. Implementation of the NHS reforms has involved a major revision of the structure, management and line of accountability of FHSAs.

The size of FHSAs has been reduced; the number of GP members was cut from seven to one. New general managers have been appointed with responsibility for managing the contractor services. In brief, the role of the FHSA has changed from administering to managing the family doctor service. At the same time LMCs have been pushed towards a more defensive 'union' type relationship with FHSAs, away from the traditional partnership role. Only time will reveal the full effect of these substantial changes.

Appendix 1: Index to the Statement of Fees and Allowances

Appendix 2: List of abbreviations

BMA	British Medical Association
BPA	Basic Practice Allowance
DHA	District Health Authority
FHSA	Family Health Services Authority
FPC	Family Practitioner Committee
GMC	General Medical Council
GMPS	General Medical and Pharmaceutical Services
GMS	General Medical Services
GMSC	General Medical Services Committee
LMC	Local Medical Committee
MMS	Maternity Medical Services
MPC	Medical Practices Committee
MSC	Medical Service Committee
NHS	National Health Service
NI	National Insurance
SCT	Service Committees and Tribunal
SFA	Statement of Fees and Allowances
SMP	Statutory Maternity Pay
SSP	Statutory Sick Pay

Appendix 3: Parliamentary regulations affecting general practice

England and Wales

General Medical Services Regulations

S.I.	Title
1992 No. 635	The NHS (GMS) Regulations 1992
1993 No. 540	The NHS (GMS) Amendment Regulations 1993

Pharmaceutical Services Regulations

S.I.	Title
1992 No. 662	The NHS (Pharmaceutical Services) Regulations 1992

Service Committees and Tribunal Regulations

S.I.	Title
1992 No. 664	The NHS (SCT) Regulations 1992

Fund-holding Practices Regulations

S.I.	Title
1990 No. 1753	The NHS (Fund-holding Practices) (Applications and Recognition) Regulations 1990
1991 No. 582	The NHS (Fund-holding Practices) (General) Regulations 1991
1992 No. 636	The NHS (Fund-holding Practices) (Amendment) Regulations 1992

Other Relevant Regulations

S.I.	Title
1979 No. 1644	The NHS (Vocational Training) Regulations 1979

S.I.	Title
1981 No. 774	The NHS (Linguistic Knowledge for General Medical Services and General Dental Services) Regulations 1981
1982 No. 288	The Health Service Act 1980 (Consequential Amendments) Order 1982
1985 No. 39	The Family Practitioner Committees (Consequential Modifications) Order 1985
1985 No. 1353	The NHS (Vocational Training) Amendment Regulations 1985
1986 No. 1642	The NHS (Vocational Training) Amendment Regulations 1986
1988 No. 866	The NHS (GMPS and Charges for Drugs) Amendment Regulations 1988
1989 No. 306	The NHS (Charges to Overseas Visitors) Regulations 1989
1989 No. 419	The NHS (Charges for Drugs and Appliances) Regulations 1989
1990 No. 537	The NHS (Charges for Drugs and Appliances) Amendment Regulations 1990
1991 No. 406	The NHS (Vocational Training) Amendment Regulations 1991
1991 No. 438	The NHS (Charges to Overseas Visitors) Amendment Regulations 1991
1991 No. 579	The NHS (Charges for Drugs and Appliances) Amendment Regulations 1991
1992 No. 365	The NHS (Charges for Drugs and Appliances) Amendment Regulations 1992
1992 No. 660	The NHS (Appellate and Other Functions) Regulations 1992

Scotland

General Medical and Pharmaceutical Regulations

S.I.	Title
1974 No. 506	The NHS (GMPS) (Scotland) Regulations 1974
1975 No. 696 (S. 114)	The NHS (GMPS) (Scotland) Amendment Regulations 1975
1976 No. 1574 (S. 126)	The NHS (GMPS) (Scotland) Amendment (No. 2) Regulations 1976

S.I.	Title
1978 No. 1762 (S. 155)	The NHS (GMPS) (Scotland) Amendment Regulations 1978
1981 No. 56 (S. 7)	The NHS (GMPS) (Scotland) Amendment Regulations 1981
1981 No. 965 (S. 95)	The NHS (GMPS) (Scotland) Amendment (No. 2) Regulations 1981
1982 No. 1279 (S. 152)	The NHS (GMPS) (Scotland) Amendment Regulations 1982
1985 No. 296 (S. 29)	The NHS (GMPS) (Scotland) Amendment Regulations 1985
1985 No. 534 (S. 51)	The NHS (GMPS) (Scotland) Amendment (No. 2) Regulations 1985
1985 No. 804 (S. 72)	The NHS (GMPS) (Scotland) Amendment (No. 3) Regulations 1985
1985 No. 1625 (S. 125)	The NHS (GMPS) (Scotland) Amendment (No. 4) Regulations 1985
1986 No. 303 (S. 22)	The NHS (GMPS) (Scotland) Amendment Regulations 1986
1986 No. 925 (S. 80)	The NHS (GMPS) (Scotland) Amendment (No. 2) Regulations 1986
1986 No. 1507 (S. 118)	The NHS (GMPS) (Scotland) Amendment (No. 3) Regulations 1986
1986 No. 2310 (S. 171)	The NHS (GMPS) (Scotland) Amendment (No. 4) Regulations 1986
1987 No. 385 (S. 35)	The NHS (GMPS) (Scotland) Amendment Regulations 1987
1987 No. 386 (S.36)	The NHS (GMPS) (Scotland) Amendment (No. 2) Regulations 1987
1987 No. 1382 (S. 102)	The NHS (GMPS) (Scotland) Amendment (No. 3) Regulations 1987

S.I.	Title
1988 No. 1073 (S. 105)	The NHS (GMPS and Charges for Drugs) (Scotland) Amendment Regulations 1988
1988 No. 1454 (S. 140)	The NHS (GMPS) (Scotland) Amendment (No. 2) Regulations 1988
1988 No. 2259 (S. 221)	The NHS (GMPS) (Scotland) Amendment (No. 3) Regulations 1988
1989 No. 1883 (S. 135)	The NHS (GMPS) (Scotland) Amendment Regulations 1989
1989 No. 1990 (S. 139)	The NHS (GMPS) (Scotland) Amendment (No. 2) Regulations 1989
1990 No. 883 (S. 116)	The NHS (GMPS) (Scotland) Amendment Regulations 1990
1990 No. 2509 (S. 211)	The NHS (GMPS) (Scotland) Amendment (No. 2) Regulations 1990
1991 No. 572 (S. 57)	The NHS (GMPS) (Scotland) Amendment Regulations 1991
1991 No. 2241 (S. 187)	The NHS (GMPS) (Scotland) Amendment (No. 2) Regulations 1991
1992 No. 191 (S. 14)	The NHS (GMPS) (Scotland) Amendment Regulations 1992
1992 No. 2401 (S. 229)	The NHS (GMPS) (Scotland) Amendment (No. 2) Regulations 1992
1992 No. 2933 (S. 240)	The NHS (GMPS) (Scotland) Amendment (No. 3) Regulations 1992
1993 No. 521 (S. 58)	The NHS (GMPS) (Scotland) Amendment Regulations 1993

Service Committees and Tribunal Regulations

S.I.	Title
1974 No. 504	The NHS (SCT) (Scotland) Regulations 1974

S.I.	Title
1974 No. 1031 (S. 88)	The NHS (SCT) (Scotland) Amendment Regulations 1974
1988 No. 878 (S. 87)	The NHS (SCT) (Scotland) Amendment Regulations 1988
1992 No. 434 (S. 48)	The NHS (SCT) (Scotland) Regulations 1992

Fund-holding Practices Regulations

S.I.	Title
1990 No. 1754 (S. 167)	The NHS (Fund-holding Practices) (Applications and Recognition) (Scotland) Regulations 1990
1991 No. 573 (S. 58)	The NHS (Fund-holding Practices) (General) (Scotland) Regulations 1991
1992 No. 2379 (S. 228)	The NHS (Fund-holding Practices) (Applications and Recognition) (Scotland) Amendment Regulations 1992
1993 No. 488 (S. 53)	The NHS (Fund-holding Practices) (Scotland) Regulations 1993

Other Relevant Regulations

S.I.	Title
1987 No. 367 (S. 30)	The NHS (Charges for Drugs and Appliances) (Scotland) Amendment Regulations 1987
1987 No. 387 (S. 37)	The NHS (Charges to Overseas Visitors) (Scotland) Amendment Regulations 1987
1988 No. 13 (S. 2)	The NHS (Charges to Overseas Visitors) (Scotland) Amendment Regulations 1988
1988 No. 365 (S. 37)	The NHS (Charges for Drugs and Appliances) (Scotland) Amendment Regulations 1988
1988 No. 462 (S. 46)	The NHS (Charges to Overseas Visitors) (Scotland) Amendment (No. 2) Regulations 1988

S.I.	Title
1989 No. 326 (S. 36)	The NHS (Charges for Drugs and Appliances) (Scotland) Regulations 1989
1989 No. 364 (S. 40)	The NHS (Charges to Overseas Visitors) (Scotland) Regulations 1989
1990 No. 468 (S. 53)	The NHS (Charges for Drugs and Appliances) (Scotland) Amendment Regulations 1990
1990 No. 787 (S. 92)	The NHS (Charges for Drugs and Appliances) (Scotland) Amendment (No. 2) Regulations 1990
1991 No. 574 (S. 59)	The NHS (Charges for Drugs and Appliances) (Scotland) Amendment Regulations 1991
1991 No. 576 (S. 61)	The NHS (Vocational Training) (Scotland) Amendment Regulations 1991
1992 No. 394 (S. 38)	The NHS (Charges for Drugs and Appliances) (Scotland) Amendment Regulations 1992
1992 No. 411 (S. 44)	The NHS (Charges to Overseas Visitors) (Scotland) Amendment Regulations 1992
1993 No. 522 (S. 59)	The NHS (Charges for Drugs and Appliances) (Scotland) Amendment Regulations 1993

Appendix 4: Amendments to the Red Book issued since 1 April 1990

SFA amendment number and date	Key changes	SFA paragraph(s)
SFA 1 March 1990	• basic practice allowance: list sizes of all partners (including any part-timers) added together to calculate average list size and then distributed according to each GP's commitment irrespective of actual number of patients (presumed to be) on an individual list	12.5
	• associate doctors: consequential amendments	24.4d, 29.3, 41.5
	• payments to practitioners who provide (out of hours) services on behalf of doctors who have opted out as at 31 March 1990	71.1e, 72.2i, 73.1, 75.1, 76.1, 82.1–3
	• correction of printing errors	
SFA 2 May 1990	• new fees and allowances based on DDRB award	1/Sch 1, 81/Sch 1
	• removal of requirement to name patients when claiming for cervical cytology targets, health promotion clinics, minor surgery sessions	28.2, 30.3, 42.5, 42.6
	• amendment of example of calculation, maximum sum payable, cervical cytology targets	28.3

	• trainee practitioner scheme:
	    trainer appeals
	    medical defence organization subscription reimbursement
		
		38.3–4
		38.6e.vi

	• premises: co-operation between professionals	51.9
	• cost rents: leasehold premises cost limits	51.50.3 51/Sch 1–2
	• improvement grants: cost limits	56/Sch 2
	• reimbursement for health authority attached staff	52.7
	• computing costs	58
	• appeals procedure where an application or claim has been refused on grounds which include the FHSA's management of its cash limited funds (i.e. practice staff, premises improvements or computer costs)	80.1–2

SFA amendment number and date	Key changes	SFA paragraph(s)
SFA 3 September 1990	• change in method of calculating target payments from an individual to a partnership list basis	1/Sch 1, 2, 25, 26, 28
SFA 4 January 1991	• trainee practitioner scheme: additional motor vehicle	1/Sch 1
	• definitions: committee, FHSA	2
	• designated areas addition: calculating average list size	14.3
	• registration fees: deferment provisions etc	23
	• night visit fee: payment of higher fee	24.4.c,d,e,f
	• temporary residents: correction of error	32.12
	• minor surgery: eligible procedures	42/Sch 1
	• dispensing doctors: fees	44/Sch 2,3
	• transitional payments	83.1–4
SFA 5 April 1991	• trainee practitioner scheme: medical defence organization subscription reimbursement	38.6e.vi
	• changes to the rural practice payments scheme	43.1–22
	• dispensing doctors: fees	44/Sch 3
	• locum payments for job sharers	47, 48, 49, 50, 62, 63, 64, 68, 69, 78
	• rent and rates scheme: amended to take account of VAT on rent and the introduction of the uniform business rate, etc.	51
	• arrangements in national emergency	79.1–3
SFA 6 May 1991	• new fees and allowances based on DDRB award	1/Sch 1, 81/Sch 1, 82
	• cost limits	51/Sch 1,2,3, 56/Sch 2
	• night visit fee – amended to remove the three month minimum period for eligibility to the higher fee	24.4f
SFA 7 July 1991	• health promotion clinics: greater flexibility in meeting the criterion for payment for approved clinics	30.2–3
	• minor surgery: carrying forward of a limited number of minor surgery procedures from one quarter to a later one	42.2–3
	payment procedures	42.6–7
	• rural practice payments	1/Sch 1, 43.20–22

SFA amendment number and date	Key changes	SFA paragraph(s)
	• dispensing doctors: fees	44/Sch 3
	• GP computer reimbursement scheme	58.1–22
SFA 8 September 1991	• trainee practitioner scheme: additional motor vehicle	1/Sch 1
	• transitional payment scheme: revised rates	83
SFA 9 October 1991	• dispensing doctors: fees	44/Sch 2
	• amendments to cost rent scheme to provide for VAT on self-supply of land	51
SFA 10 April 1992	• trainee practitioner scheme: maternity leave and pay arrangements	38.32 a–d
	• supply of drugs and appliances: Prescription Pricing Division, Wales	44
	• locum allowance during confinement	49.3
	• consolidation of the GMPS Regulations 1974	
	• maternity medical services: responsibilities of practitioners and criteria for admission to obstetric list transferred to Regulations	31/Sch 1,2
SFA 11 May 1992	• new fees and allowances based on DDRB award	1/Sch 1, 81/Sch 1, 82
	• transitional payments scheme: ended on 31 March 1992	83
SFA 12 May 1992	• changes to course organizers' pay	38.5k
	• higher night visit fee to be paid when a GP sees his or her own or a partner's patients whilst working for a commercial deputizing service or large rota, and also when the creation of a job share would result in an existing rota of 10 or less breaking the 10 doctor limit	24.4
SFA13 August 1992	• trainee practitioner scheme: additional motor vehicle	1/Sch 1
	• seniority allowance: service with Foreign and Commonwealth Office in Warsaw, Moscow, Dhaka, New Delhi	16.13–14
	• health promotion clinics: moratorium	30.1–10
	• trainee practitioner scheme: removal expenses	38.7–23
	• cost limits	51.52.10–13, 51/Sch 1–3, 56/Sch 2
SFA 14 February 1993	• seniority allowance: compulsory retirement at 70	16.6–7

SFA amendment number and date	Key changes	SFA paragraph(s)
	• *Haemophilus influenzae b* (Hib) vaccine item-of-service fee	27/Sch 1
		38/Sch 2
	• trainee practitioner scheme: allowances London Weighting	1/Sch 1
	• computer costs: continuation of scheme	58.1
	• maternity medical services: change in definition of stillbirth	31.4, 31.10, 31.11

Appendix 5: Index to The National Health Service (General Medical Services) Regulations 1992

Note: References preceded by A are to the National Health Service (General Medical Services) Amendment Regulations 1993. All references are to Schedules and/or paragraphs; e.g. Sch 2/18–26 is Schedule 2, paragraphs 18 to 26.

Index